CUT
GUT

Thank you for your support
of Cut Gut Organization
and enjoy the book!

Jamie J Palfrey

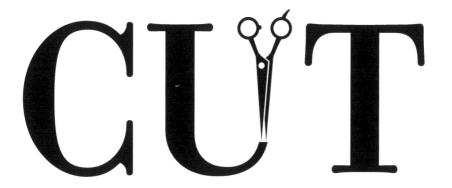

CUT

Why **Bariatric Surgery**
Could Be Right for You
Yes, *You!*

GUT

Jamie J. Palfrey, M.Ed.

Three Hearts
publishing

Published by Three Hearts Publishing

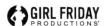

Edited and designed by Girl Friday Productions
www.girlfridayproductions.com

Cover and interior design: Rachel Marek
Editorial: Alexander Rigby, Simone Gorrindo, Naomi Burns, Lois Baron

ISBN (paperback): 978-1-7343117-0-9
ISBN (hardcover): 978-1-7343117-2-3
ISBN (ebook): 978-1-7343117-1-6

I would like to dedicate this book to my sister, Jody, who fought hard and believed that a healthy life was possible for me, even when I had given up on myself. And to my life partner, Gary, who has seen me through years of diet failures and continued to love and support me through it all. Their love gave me the strength and courage to seek out a weight-loss option that has truly saved my life. I would also like to thank my children, Gabriella and Liam, who continuously inspire me through their own perseverance in the face of life's challenges; my mother, who opened my mind to the possibility of a new path; and my entire family for their love, understanding, and support during my journey through bariatric surgery. And a big thank-you to Dr. W, whose brilliant mind, skillful hands, and caring heart have helped me live a happy, healthy life.

CONTENTS

AUTHOR'S NOTE

In recent years, people have started trending away from dieting for weight loss. For those of us at 35+ BMI or 30+ BMI with comorbid conditions, are we finally tired of trying diets that fail? It's time to have a new conversation.

I wrote this book because I want bariatric surgery to take its rightful place as a mainstream solution for substantial, sustainable, and life-changing weight loss.

FOREWORD

For decades, we've accepted the idea that obesity, regardless of the cause or degree, is a condition that results from poor self-control. And if you found yourself struggling with your weight, the problem could be eliminated by the simple act of eating less and exercising more. After a dozen years as a bariatric surgeon, I've come to one important conclusion about weight gain and obesity: it is much more complicated than we've ever believed. The factors that are responsible for obesity extend well beyond our nutritional choices. Weight gain and obesity are the result of our life's experience; they are the result of a complicated interplay between our genetics, our environment, our medical history, and even the nutritional health of our mother while we were in utero.

For some, the journey to weight loss is a difficult one, and diet and exercise are simply not enough. I believe that bariatric surgery is an excellent option for people who have struggled for years to achieve and maintain a healthy weight. The last decade has resulted in a remarkable improvement in the safety of bariatric surgery to the point that it is now being offered as an outpatient surgery. We've also completely transformed our understanding of the mechanism of these surgeries. In the past, we aligned the mechanism of bariatric surgery with our view of the cause of obesity. We assumed that these surgeries "blocked" us from eating too much or from absorbing the calories we eat. We described this mechanism almost as a suitable punishment for a lifetime of poor self-control. We now recognize that bariatric surgery primarily exerts its effects not by anatomical changes but instead though the neurohormonal changes that are induced by the surgical rearrangement of the intestines. This revolutionary finding has transformed our understanding of obesity and bariatric surgery.

Having a healthy skepticism regarding any surgical procedure is a good thing. I always encourage people to do their due diligence, to ask questions and look at the evidence, and to interview doctors and seek out other patients to compare notes. The societal stigma surrounding obesity is real, and I have heard many heartbreaking stories over the years from patients. So too is the stigma around bariatric surgery as a treatment for metabolic disease.

This is why I am so happy to see this book on bariatric surgery, written from the patient's perspective. Jamie J. Palfrey can attest to the experience of being an obese person and the efficacy of this surgery better than any doctor because she has lived it. Her story—her weight gain despite her healthy lifestyle; her attempts to lose weight through diet, exercise, and medication; and the overt and covert reproach from friends and strangers—is all too common. Thankfully, she was able to sort through the old narratives and outdated information that maintain the myth of obesity as a personal failing. Once she recognized her situation as a real medical condition, the real work began.

It is time to start recognizing that obesity is a disease of fat storage, not a symptom of weak willpower or lack of discipline. It is time for us to start looking at obesity objectively, to break free of shame. We are blessed to live in a time when a real medical treatment exists for obesity, and I hope that as more patients come forward and share their stories, it will become accepted as the effective weight-loss tool that it is. *Cut Gut: Why Bariatric Surgery Could Be Right for You—Yes, You!* represents a critical step in the right direction.

Matthew Weiner, MD, author of *A Pound of Cure: Change Your Eating and Your Life, One Step at a Time* and *How Weight Loss Surgery Really Works: And How to Make It Work for You*

INTRODUCTION

You did it. You're here. You picked up this book because you're tired of being overweight. Obese. Fat. Call it whatever you like. The point is that you have excess weight, and you've been lugging those pounds around for a long time now. You've tried all the diets. Read all the books. Endured all the pills, supplements, regimens, gyms, and boot camps. Maybe you even gave it your all on *The Biggest Loser*. You've tried everything, and you've failed. But maybe you haven't tried *everything*. Maybe, just maybe, you're ready to try something different. Something substantial. Something sustaining. Something revolutionary.

I used to be in your shoes. But now, in my early fifties, I'm thin. Why? Because I decided to do something next-level and have bariatric surgery. After thirty years of exercising and dieting and medicating, I hit a brick wall. I saw a TV show about a 600-pound person who underwent gastric bypass and was now at a healthy weight. My initial thoughts were, *Well, that is for the severely overweight. I only need to lose 80 pounds. This 80 freaking pounds that I've been hauling around for 30 years!* Then, for a moment, I let myself consider it. *Maybe?* I thought. Then, *Nah . . . surgery is not for me. They're going to rearrange my guts. What?! Nope. That's crazy. What if it doesn't work? What if something goes wrong? What if . . .*

I resigned myself then and there to staying fat. I was tired of trying and always failing. I said to myself, *This is just you. You are always going to be this way.* But then I asked myself, *What might happen if I don't try surgery? Will I become diabetic? Will my ticker give out? Will I have to use a walker when I'm sixty? Will I need a shopping cart scooter to get around the grocery store?*

I labored over the pros and cons for a long time. I considered my family and my quality of life. And after I'd written it all down, the pros far outweighed the cons. I wanted to live and be comfortable in my body, to be released from worrying about my poor little heart beating away in my chest, my swollen ankles, and the host of other health concerns that come with being overweight. And I definitely didn't want to face the social stigmas associated with being overweight. I was no longer concerned with perfection (gracing the cover of *Shape* magazine was not my goal). I just wanted to live well.

So I pulled the trigger and got bariatric surgery. I only wish I'd done it sooner.

In no way do I want to demonize fatness. I know as well as anyone that for many of us, obesity is the hand we were dealt. It took me many years to realize that obesity is neither morally good nor morally bad. I'm so glad to see that the younger generation is changing the conversation around weight and that people, particularly women, are pushing back against not just body shaming but also the idea that appearance is the most important marker of our worth. My hope is that, as the taboo surrounding fatness loses its power, we can address the issue itself directly, without the shame and blame, the secrecy, and the self-flagellation. If we as a society stop judging obesity as a character flaw, stop assuming that all obese people somehow deserve to be fat, we can talk openly about its health implications, especially those that come about as we grow older: diabetes, high blood pressure, coronary heart disease, and physical pain—real issues that require real treatment.

This is not a diet or self-help book but a mix of my story and the practical information I've learned along the way through years of research. To be clear, I am not a doctor or a dietician, and I don't own a medical facility or a gastric band–supply company. The only thing I'm trying to sell here is the idea that bariatric surgery is an option worth considering. It is not just a Hail Mary reserved for the super obese.

I am walking proof that bariatric surgery can positively and indelibly change a person's life. Unfortunately, few have considered this treatment. I'm not surprised. In my opinion, there are not enough mainstream educational resources on bariatric surgery. And many insurance plans don't cover it. Even those that do often come with arduous qualifying processes and significant out-of-pocket costs. Then there are those who can't afford health insurance to begin with. That's why I created Cut Gut Organization, a nonprofit devoted to raising money to help those who could benefit from the surgery and need some financial and educational assistance to make it happen.

Throughout my adult life, I've obsessively researched all angles of the weight-gain phenomenon, and I can tell you that both science and popular opinion on the subject are constantly changing. In the 1990s, "fat free" was the thing; in the 2010s, fat and high-fat meal plans like the ketogenic diet are hailed as veritable cure-alls. The pendulum is always swinging, and on top of that, every day someone is promoting a brand-new methodology or exercise program—or giving an old one a face-lift.

I've done my best to present solid information from reputable sources in this book. I am a business professional, not a doctor, a scientist, or an academic. I am offering the perspective of the patient, someone who lived for many years with a metabolic malady and then underwent a medical intervention that changed everything. In this book you will find an exploration of why some of us are fat no matter how hard we try to lose weight; what it means to live as a fat person in a society that shames fat people; how the diet and pharmaceutical industries help some and hurt others; everything you need to know if you're considering taking the far-from-painless step toward bariatric surgery; and how to live life again once you've had your guts cut.

I hope this book helps you understand the social phenomenon of fatness better, gives you practical information about bariatric surgery, points you in the direction of medical associations and other resources that can educate you further, and supports you in your health and wellness journey. More than anything, I hope this book is a vital step toward finding a lasting solution for the 1.9 billion adults in the world who are currently overweight and, within this group, the 650 million obese individuals who struggle with a 30+ body mass index (BMI), many with comorbidity conditions. This book is for those who have had every diet and exercise routine they've ever tried fail them. Yes, they failed you—not the other way around.

After reading this, I want you to feel brave instead of ashamed, hopeful rather than pessimistic, empowered, and no longer enslaved. I hope this book fills you with the sense that you are not alone and that you have powerful, effective, and legitimate tools in your tool belt that can help you achieve the health and longevity you've been seeking for so long.

PART
ONE

CHAPTER 1

Cut Loose

Time is a precious thing. Never waste it.
—Willy Wonka, *Willy Wonka & the Chocolate Factory*

Cut Throat

I must have been one of the most photographed babies in all of history. Born at 6 pounds 4 ounces, I was a healthy infant, neither too big nor too small. "Just right." My mom, an elementary school teacher, liked to dress me up in frilly dresses and, as I came into toddlerhood, style my hair in perfect ringlets, then smudge on a dash of lipstick and give my cheeks a pinch before whipping out the camera. Later she would sew us matching dresses and enter us in mother-daughter look-alike beauty pageants. Beaver Cleaver, anyone? Exactly.

I was born stereotypically "Barbie pretty," an all-American girl with bright blue eyes and shiny blonde hair. Arriving in this world with looks that our society venerates was simply a stroke of genetic luck, like having a naturally good ear for music or a way with numbers. I was treated like a little princess, and by kindergarten, I was one of the popular kids, with a slew of boys that "liked" me and a crew made up of other popular little girls. But it wasn't just my peers that noticed me—older kids and adults, family friends, and total strangers seemed to take an interest in me too. Some innocently oohed and aahed over my neatly styled hair or fancy new dress, while others seemed so taken with my looks, their interest verged on the lecherous.

I developed early, and by second grade, I was wearing a bra and eliciting a kind of attention that I neither wanted nor understood. Elementary classmates made fun of the bra outline they could see under my shirt (as I was the only girl wearing one), and some were bold enough to run up behind me and snap my bra straps and then run away laughing. I noticed that some teenagers and adults were not looking me in the eye but instead looking at my body as they talked to me. The stares and wide smiles made me feel uncomfortable and isolated.

By junior high, it seemed as if everyone had an opinion about how I looked and, more importantly, felt free to share it with me. In gym class, we were required to jog, and some of the boys, who themselves had just entered the awkwardness of puberty, would yell, "Watch out or you'll get a black eye!" as my very large boobs bobbled around on my tiny frame. (Unfortunately, my adolescent years arrived prior to the invention of decent sports bras.) I felt as if a spotlight was on me wherever I went. It was both a blessing and a curse.

My junior high and high school, like many people's, were cutthroat and competitive environments. Movies like *Mean Girls* are a bona fide depiction of what life back then was like for me. I was uncomfortable in my own skin. At seventeen years old and 123 pounds, I felt horribly overweight, perpetually tugging on my purposely baggy clothes to hide my hourglass figure.

If I could go back in time, I would tell that girl to stop fidgeting. Stop adjusting her shirt, smoothing her hair, and covertly checking her reflection in any semi-reflective surface. The amount of energy I spent trying to conceal my imagined imperfections! My self-consciousness came, in part, from my ballet training, cheer-leading practices, and modeling lessons, where my teachers' and coaches' judgment of my body was explicit. In part, simply being a teenager was to blame—I swear, you could not pay me enough to go through that life phase again! Add to that being female in this world. I don't think it's breaking news to say that people look at girls and women and tend to make—and freely share—judgments on our appearances.

In this time-machine scenario, I'd also tell that girl, "Enjoy it while you can" in that annoying, patronizing way that older people boss adolescents. I was young and energetic. I spent my time hiking and biking and swimming and horseback riding and playing competitive racquetball and doing aerobics at the local gym, but I had no damn idea that this was a shining moment, that I would never again feel so good and able in my body. In short, I was your typical teenage nightmare, golden and popular, outwardly self-assured but incredibly insecure.

It wasn't until I left home for college that I began to gain unwanted weight. Like so many college freshmen, I found those first few months away from home disorienting. I was lonely and homesick, trying to navigate classes that were way harder than the ones I'd taken in high school, impress a slew of strangers enough for them to become my friends, and figure out what it meant to take care of myself without any parental oversight. My mom and dad had run our house like clock-work, with a wholesome homemade dinner on the table every night at 6:00 p.m. I inherited a sweet tooth from my dad, who believed a meal couldn't be digested properly without a piece of chocolate as a "chaser." Beyond those desserts and the rare walks with my best girlfriend to 7-Eleven, where I'd blow my allowance on Cup-o-Gold candy bars and cream soda, I grew up with a healthy and regular diet, in a loving and regular family. Throughout my childhood, I had a "normal" relation-ship with food.

In college, all that went out the window. All of a sudden, the cafe-teria offered a seemingly endless supply of sweets and no one telling me I had to finish my peas before I could be excused from the table. For someone with an overactive sweet tooth, this was a dream come true, like walking into my own personal Willy Wonka's Chocolate Factory. During that stressful first year away from home, I turned toward sweets for comfort. At breakfast I ate blueberry muffins and sugar-dusted scones to my heart's content. Lunchtime meant trips to the self-serve soda fountain and cookies of every stripe, from chocolate chip to peanut butter to oatmeal raisin. And on those nights when I was feeling particularly stressed or anxious or overwhelmed, ice cream and cake after dinner were my saving grace. Eating junk food was a way of life at college: cheese-smothered macaroni, bland Chinese food, spicy chicken wings, and potatoes and gravy. And of course, I'd indulge in pizza at the local pizza joint with friends, followed by contraband beer back at the dorms. Though my sweet-tooth rampage didn't last longer than a few semesters, this was just enough time for the freshman fifteen to turn into the sophomore spread.

If you're thinking to yourself, *Of course you gained weight. With a diet like that, you have no one to blame but yourself!* Well, you aren't exactly wrong. For me, eating junk equals gaining weight. I was certainly not alone among my peers in eating my feelings or exploring my newfound gastronomic freedom, but many of my friends' metabolisms powered through this behavior. A friend of mine from Northern California who had been raised without sugar or meat ate nothing but Lucky Charms and Taco Bell for a year straight when he got to college. Another busy friend would forget to eat all day and then fit about five meals' worth of pizza into single epic late-night binges. For all of us, beer flowed like, well, beer. Yet I was one of the few students who seemed to be packing on extra weight.

Perhaps you were the rare virtuous soul who got through college on the daily three square meals, but I'll bet if you ask around, you'll find that most of your friends weren't so disciplined. So even though I might have drained too many Solo cups and snarfed too many cupcakes, most of my friends did the same. Some people, like me, paid the price on the scale, and many didn't. Even after I steered my tray away from the dessert table and exchanged the mac and cheese for salad and lean protein, the weight I had gained stuck. From freshman year of college on, I gained weight in spurts over time, never really understanding how or why, even though my overall eating and exercise habits had generally returned to the same healthy ones my parents had instilled in me before college.

Though I didn't know it at the time, I was coming into a new set point during my college years. No, I'm not referring to a tennis score. I'm talking about Set Point Theory, which postulates that the body has a natural weight range that it fights to return to. In 1953, a scientist by the name of G. C. Kennedy experimented on some rats and came up with a model of body fat regulation upon which Set Point Theory is based. In his model, our body fat produces a signal that regulates food intake and energy expenditure. Simply put, the more fat you have, the less hungry and more energized you should be, and vice versa. It turns out though that, for some, this metabolic feedback loop can get broken (I will discuss this further later in this chapter).

I reached my maximum weight of 238 pounds at age thirty-seven, and grew accustomed to another kind of attention, one that was familiar but had a different heat to it. It no longer felt like admiration or appreciation—often it was downright unfriendly. In my youth, people had liked me for something I had little control over; now, in my adulthood, people disliked me for the same. Of course, they—and I—thought I had control over it. I think if there'd been a poll, we would have all agreed that my fatness was a symbol of my failure or, more specifically, of my moral failing. Even though all my hard work to lose weight proved otherwise, I had internalized the belief that fat people earned their fatness through ignorance, poor decision-making, and laziness, and so they deserved those sidelong glances and disapproving stares. "Pretty girl," I could practically hear them thinking. "Such a shame she's let herself get fat."

A Growing Gut

Rat experiments are one thing; real-life human experience is quite another. Walk around any shopping mall or look out over the stands at a baseball game in America, and it'll become hard to argue that our fat regulation systems are doing their job. In fact, almost 40 percent of adult Americans are now considered obese, which the National Institute of Health classifies as having a body mass index, or BMI, of 30 or higher (I'll talk more about BMI in the upcoming sections). By contrast, Americans are considered overweight if they have a BMI of 25–29.9 and are classified as "normal" if their BMI falls between 18.5 and 24.9.

There are a whole lot of variables that contribute to obesity in America, including issues with funding for public school physical education, access to medical care, and availability of nutrient-dense food. Not everyone has a natural foods co-op in their neighborhood, and even if they do, fresh-pressed carrot-celery-ginger juice costs a lot more than a slushy at the gas station convenience store. Still, for every obese person eating a cardboard dish of garlic fries at the Mariners' game, there is a thin person doing the same. So why is it that some people who occasionally indulge maintain an unhealthy weight of 240 pounds, while others couldn't hit 100 pounds soaking wet if they tried and others tip the scales at 600 pounds? The simple answer is, it is not simple. The even simpler answer is, I don't think we quite know.

In his Set Point Theory of Weight, Kennedy postulates that your set point is (1) the weight at which your body is programmed to func-tion optimally *and* (2) the weight that your body will fight to maintain. Expanding, then, on the Set Point Theory of Weight, I believe the set point metabolic feedback loop stops functioning properly during what I call "breakthrough episodes." In these episodes, your body breaks through your current set point and moves to a new higher weight set point. There are genetic, hormonal (epigenetic), and environmental components involved in this process, an infuriating Gordian knot of nature versus nurture.

We don't know exactly why some people gain weight easily and struggle to lose it. However, many experts agree that the creation of a new set point can be due to a variety of factors, including overeating, stress, lack of sleep, hormones, medication, injury, or illness. Having a baby. Going on a bender. Taking a new antidepressant. Grieving for a lost loved one. The list goes on, and encapsulates what is otherwise known as "being human." I like to think of the body's set point as the Wonkavator, the glass elevator at the end of the original *Willy Wonka & the Chocolate Factory* from 1971. I refer to these "being human" events as "Wonkavator rides" that our bodies take.

Imagine you are in the Wonkavator with a wild-eyed, top-hatted Gene Wilder, gentle Grandpa, and gold-hearted Charlie, careening toward the glass ceiling. "Hold on everybody, here it comes!" Willy Wonka yells as the elevator breaks through, and your fear turns into awe as "Pure Imagination" plays in the background. Instead of getting cut to ribbons by shattered glass, you are intact, and the elevator is floating, going higher and higher with no particular destination. What fun!

Except, remember, we're using the Wonkavator as an analogy for set point. In this analogy, the free float is your weight, climbing higher and higher. Eventually it will land, but where? It may land at the same level as the original launch site, like a regular elevator returning to the lobby. But it could settle just a little ways up, say, 5 feet (or 5 pounds). Or maybe it settles a little further, at 20 feet (or 20 pounds) on a green hillside. Or perhaps it lands 100 pounds up on a cold, windblown mountain. Wherever it lands, there you are. This is your new home— your new set point—and life builds up around it.

Let's say you were 150 pounds and a back injury forced you into two months of bed rest and some serious emotional eating, causing you to gain weight. Now you are on the mend and your regular more healthy eating habits have returned, but instead of your body fighting to quickly return you to your 150-pound set point, it has landed you at 170 pounds, and your body now accepts this new weight as the new normal. In this two-month breakthrough episode, your set point has gone from 150 to 170 pounds, and it is here, at this higher weight, that your body will now fight to stay, barring further unforeseen events. But if life is famous for one thing, it's unforeseen events. So, a few years later, you find yourself strapped in for another potential Wonkavator ride with Charlie, Grandpa, and Willy Wonka. The question is now, will you return to that cozy set point spot of 170 pounds on the hillside? Or will you break through your set point and find residence higher up the mountain?

For those of us who have a set point that tends to adjust upward, this is no thrill ride; it's straight terror, particularly when you realize that you have *little to no control* over where you land. When some men get older and their testosterone levels drop, their hair falls out, regardless of their diet, exercise habits, or choice of shampoo. As other men get older, their weight climbs, regardless of diet, exercise, or expensive weight-loss supplements. Some people just get bald. Some people just get fat. It's because of genes. It's because of hormones. It's because of environment. It's because life's not fair.

At whatever new set point you land—190 pounds, 220 pounds, 400 pounds—your brain now believes this is where you are supposed to be, the best weight for you to sustain life. In other words, if you then try to go below that weight, your body is going to fight to get you back to your new set point. People who have gained weight then lost it through extreme dieting often gain it back not because they got lazy and decided to piss it all away but because hunger is a primal sensation and eating is a primal behavior created for the sake of survival. Your set point is a powerful thing, and your body will pull out all the stops to ensure it is maintained.

Perhaps you're asking yourself how in the world your brain could believe that hauling around an extra 50 or 150 pounds is an optimal state of affairs. But think about it: it wasn't until very recently that humans had access to an essentially unlimited supply of high-energy foods. Before eating hot dogs was a competitive sport, humans didn't always know where their next meal would be coming from, and they had to do a lot more than pull up to the drive-through window to get it. Had I been alive back then, my tendency toward fat storage would have given me a significant advantage over my skinny brothers and sisters. You might even say that those of us who more easily pack on the pounds are evolutionarily superior—or at least we were up until the twenty-four-hour drive-through availability of the 770-calorie Double Quarter Pounder and 730-calorie Butterfinger Blizzard became a fact of life. "The Caveman's Curse," an article published by the *Economist* in 2012, aptly points out that during the Paleolithic era, a body's ability to store excess fat was a survival advantage.

If I carefully examine my own history, I can identify specific times that I pushed my set point too far. Of course, I wasn't trying to do this, nor was I even aware that a breakthrough episode was happening. Those two semesters that I carbo-loaded in my college cafeteria was my very first breakthrough episode: instead of losing the weight as many of my friends did (or never gaining any in the first place), the extra pounds stuck around. Why did my body give up the fight to return my elevator to the lobby? I'll probably never know.

The bursts of weight gain continued as I went through other life transitions and phases: getting married, having children, and holding down a demanding job. Meanwhile, my husband, who is one of these annoying people who can still fit in the tux he wore to senior prom, matched my lifestyle (minus the pregnancies), yet I alone suffered the long-term consequences of eating a bowl of movie-night popcorn. While he does take good care of himself, he's not a fundamentalist about it. Over the years there have been a couple of times that he has gained up to 20 pounds, but his body always returns him effortlessly to his original set point. This has led me to the conclusion that he has lucked into a solid set point that is seemingly resistant to breakthrough episodes and allows for some temporary weight-gain elasticity, while my body has always seemed ready and willing to go on Wonkavator rides, settling on higher and higher ground.

BREAKTHROUGH EPISODE
"WONKAVATOR RIDE"

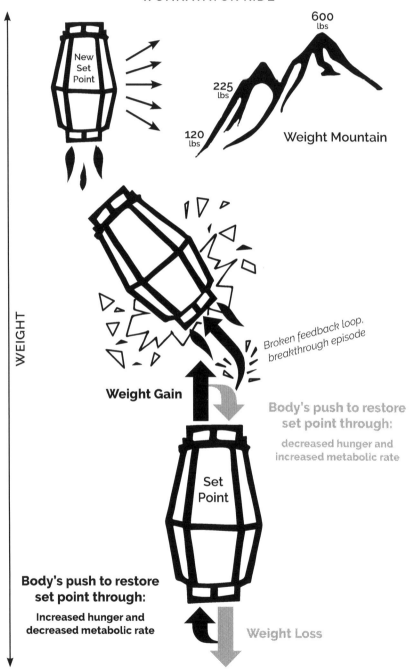

New Set Point

600 lbs

225 lbs

120 lbs

Weight Mountain

Broken feedback loop, breakthrough episode

Weight Gain

Body's push to restore set point through:
decreased hunger and increased metabolic rate

Set Point

WEIGHT

Body's push to restore set point through:
Increased hunger and decreased metabolic rate

Weight Loss

Gut Hormones and Your Appetite

I am a die-hard dog person, so I like to think about body/metabolic type in doggie terms. Take two of my dogs, for example: English bulldogs. These dogs are medium sized and thick. No matter how much you starve them or run them, they will never, ever become whippets. No matter how much you feed them and let them sit around all day on the couch, they will never, ever become Great Danes (I also have two of those). They will always be English bulldogs, and though, like humans, they can lose and gain weight, they have a set range. The skinniest English bulldog will always weigh more than the burliest whippet, and even the most obese bulldog will never weigh as much as the daintiest Great Dane.

It's the same for humans. We come in all shapes and sizes, which are determined by genes as well as environment. Someone with a skeletal structure designed by the DNA gods to max out at 5 feet 6 will never reach 6 feet 6, despite dietary efforts and NBA dreams; someone with curly hair can marshal an army of chemicals to straighten it, but the jig is up the minute she gets caught in the rain. Our metabolic types differ in much the same way, and in the same way, we have only so much control. For some, set point remains relatively stable over a lifetime. These very lucky few can gain 5 pounds at Christmas and lose them by mid-January, or get rid of the baby weight by the time little Grace cuts her first tooth. For some, it's a matter of strict diet and exercise; for others, it's relatively effortless. If you've struggled with your weight, you are probably all too aware of those jerks who seem to live on a diet of cheeseburgers and never gain an ounce. (Of course, there are other health issues to be concerned about with such a diet.) I'll admit, I've had more than one murderous thought about my friend Aaliyah, who loves pasta and hates cardio and never tips the scale past 120. Then there are those other folks, such as myself, who merely think about a slice of pizza and gain 3 pounds. We are the ones with the more easily broken metabolic feedback loop.

As I see it, adults could be grouped into four metabolic categories:

- **Cemented Celia:** This is a person (like my husband) whose set point is firmly cemented. These people possess an extraordinary metabolic mechanism that enables them to maintain a general weight/set point, regardless of their dietary and activity changes.
- **Sticky Stanley:** This person's set point generally "sticks" around. Their set point will experience a breakthrough episode if pushed really hard, but they can rely on it to stay strong and hold steady throughout their adult life.
- **Loosey Larry:** This is a person (like me) whose set point is irritatingly "loose in the saddle" and ready to go on a Wonkavator ride after a mere weekend of Super Bowl parties involving too many hot dogs, hamburgers, potato chips, margaritas, and cookies.
- **Flying Freda:** Poor Freda has whiplash from a never-ending nonlinear (up, down, and sideways) Wonkavator ride! This person's set point is so ever changing that the term *set point* may be a misnomer. While we know that our bodies need a set point at which to maintain life, this person's metabolism is so broken that their weight has been flying around the scale for years, seemingly never landing in one place.

Obviously, if we understood the glitches in Loosey Larry's and Flying Freda's metabolisms, we would have fixed them long ago. But metabolism and metabolic disease are still essentially a black box, though the medical field is making new discoveries about them every day. What we do know is that our metabolisms are regulated by a soup of different hormones, including cortisol, insulin, peptide YY, and neuropeptide Y, as well as the hunger and satiety hormones ghrelin, leptin, glucagon-like peptide-1, and cholecystokinin.

Again, let me reiterate that I am not a doctor or medical scientist and that theories of the human body are amended all the time.

Remember, it wasn't all that long ago that physicians stopped using leeches as a panacea; likewise, in the beginning of 2019, a formerly illegal party drug known as Special K was approved by the FDA (in a modified form) as an antidepressant. That being said, the following discussion is based on what I've found through countless hours of reading medical journals and white papers, watching documentaries, interviewing dozens of metabolic physicians and patients, and living with metabolic disease. My hope here is to present my current understanding of metabolism in a way that makes sense to other nondoctors and nonmedical scientists. I am aiming to be your translator, your messenger.

The two leading hunger hormones, ghrelin and leptin, were recently discovered in the 1990s. Since I have declared war on ghrelin, I often refer to it as "ghrrrelin." When I think of it, I imagine myself as Xena, Warrior Princess, hollering as I ride horseback into battle in an iron-and-leather bustier. It is known as "the hunger hormone" because it works to increase your appetite and encourages fat storage. It is secreted primarily through your stomach lining, though small amounts of it are also found in your small intestine, pancreas, and brain. Once released, ghrelin finds its way into your blood and crosses the blood-brain barrier, where its signals go directly to the hypothalamus, an almond-shaped region in the middle of the brain. To greatly simplify a very complex physiological process, ghrelin tells you when to be hungry. It also has protective effects on the cardiovascular system, such as decreasing blood pressure, and plays a role in the control of insulin by suppressing glucose-stimulated insulin secretion.

In a normally functioning body system, ghrelin is highest when your stomach is empty and lowest when you have just eaten. But in obese people, this metabolic process is sometimes broken, resulting in a greater and more continuous release of ghrelin in their bodies, even when they've just eaten. To add insult to injury, in the process of gaining weight, we physically stretch out our stomachs from excess food intake, thereby expanding the stomach lining, which allows even more ghrelin to be produced! And if we drastically restrict our calorie intake and swing to the other side of the pendulum, our body reacts by creating a spike in ghrelin in order to maintain its current weight/set point. Basically, for fat people, it's often a damned-if-you-do-damned-if-you-don't situation. Scientists are working to uncover more information about the relationship between obesity and ghrelin by studying the high-circulating ghrelin levels in people with Prader-Willi syndrome, who are often severely obese. Prader-Willi syndrome is a genetic disorder that causes constant hunger, often leading to overeating and complications like obesity, heart disease, and type 2 diabetes, among other behavioral, intellectual, and physical problems. I wish these scientists Godspeed in their quest for information.

The second leading hunger hormone is leptin, which I affectionately call "lovely leptin." When I think of leptin, violins play and a bevy of swans take flight. This hormone works in the opposite way that ghrelin does. It is made by fat and secreted into the circulatory system, then travels to the hypothalamus, where it relays the message that you have enough fat and, through complex signals, stifles hunger. In a perfect metabolic world, the more body fat you have, the more leptin you will secrete and the less hungry you'll be; the less fat you have, the less leptin you'll produce and the hungrier you will be.

HUNGER HORMONES

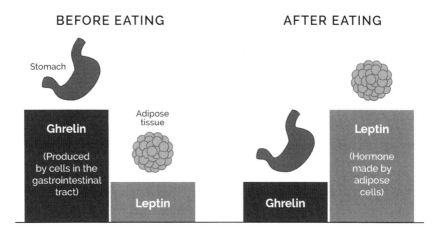

BEFORE EATING   AFTER EATING

You might be thinking, *All you need is a big dose of leptin and the pounds will just evaporate!* When leptin was discovered in 1994, scientists did indeed think they'd hit the jackpot after it was successfully injected into obese mice to make them lose weight. They'd finally found the miracle cure! All they needed to do was to develop a leptin pill for humans and—voilà!—the weight would drop off and the money would start rolling in. Unfortunately, scientists subsequently discovered that lovely leptin works only on mice (and people) that already have genetically deficient leptin levels, a small subset of the population at approximately 3 percent. For the other 97 percent of us, we could inject buckets of leptin straight into our veins and it would not help us lose any weight.

That's because the problem isn't that our natural leptin levels aren't high enough; it's that, over time, we can become leptin resistant. Leptin resistance is similar to insulin resistance in that the body and brain have stopped "communicating" or adequately receiving signals. Multiple studies have found that obese people's brains just aren't listening to leptin's signals and that, for them, leptin release doesn't result in a drop in appetite or an increase in metabolic function.

There are many unanswered questions about how and why a resistance to leptin occurs in some people who have excess fat. One theory is that leptin can't get to the hypothalamus because the proteins that transport it across the blood-brain barrier (which is a filtering mechanism of the capillaries that carry blood to the brain and spinal cord tissue, blocking the passage of certain substances) aren't working. Researchers made this postulation when they discovered a buildup of leptin was found in the cerebral spinal fluid, sitting idly by instead of sending messages to the hypothalamus. Another theory is that overweight people experience a mutation of the leptin receptor, meaning that even if leptin's important message arrives, there's no one there to answer the door.

While much more research is still needed to understand the processes that control hunger, digestion, and metabolism, the following (vastly simplified) graphic offers a general primer on these complex chemical mechanisms in our bodies.

LEPTIN RESISTANCE AND WEIGHT-GAIN CYCLE

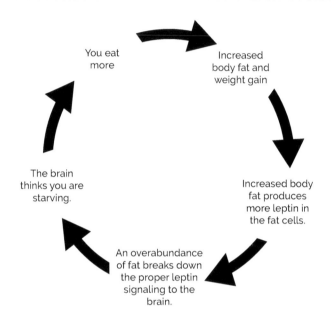

When you go below your body's established set point, whether you are in the normal range of weight or are obese, ghrelin (and other hormones) works to increase appetite (sometimes uncontrollably) and metabolism adjusts downward to try to return you quickly to that weight. Your metabolism may slow down to the point that you feel fatigued and nearly unable to perform your regular activities, let alone meet your workout partner at the gym. In the same vein, the opposite chemical reaction will occur if you go above your set point. The body will use leptin (and other chemicals) to try to fight against the weight gain by increasing its metabolic rate and lowering hunger to try to burn off the unwanted calories. Unless, of course, your ghrelin and leptin signals aren't working properly. Then, instead of losing the weight, your body resets the set point.

So who or what is responsible for all of your weight gain? Should we blame *you*, as most of society does? Should we blame a metabolic disease, broken set point, and haywire hormones? Should we assume you've tried every diet, drug, and exercise program with no lasting results? Should we assume you've let your weight and health spin out of control and you've done little or nothing about it? Does it even matter who or what is responsible? It does, and here's why:

If you've diligently tried dieting and exercise over and over again, and your weight has yo-yoed and you have been unable to achieve a lasting normal BMI, it is likely your metabolic function is not working correctly and is fighting you every step of the way. If this scenario rings true for you, it tells me that you have shown the discipline and willingness (at least at times) to make lifestyle changes in order to improve your health but have so far been unsuccessful at maintaining them.

It would be remiss of me, however, to blame everything on a broken metabolism. Stress eating, long periods of continuous poor food choices, and a sedentary lifestyle are something we must take responsibility for if we hope to make permanent changes after bariatric surgery. You still have to make the choice to pick up a handful of almonds as a snack rather than potato chips. If you rely on the initial food restriction post-surgery without fundamentally changing your eating habits, you will regain some unwanted weight. The key is, it becomes infinitely easier to make these changes post-surgery due to your brain's new ability to recognize that you are overfed and overweight.

Gauging Your Gut with BMI

When I was at my highest set point of 238 pounds, my body mass index (BMI) was 39. BMI is a commonly used calculation that takes into account the basic dimensions of height and weight and spits out a number. This is an imperfect system that is meant to help people assess their size in order to address underlying or potential health problems and outcomes. But everyone does not fit neatly into a box with a pretty red bow tied around it to be delivered to the Statistics Gods.

Keep that in mind as I state some generalities about how our health relates to our BMIs. If you don't know your BMI, you can calculate it using the many available online tools. (I like the one through the National Heart, Lung, and Blood Institute website.) Note that your BMI doesn't necessarily have anything to do with how you *feel* or *behave*, and it definitely has nothing to do with whether you are a good person. It doesn't necessarily have bearing on your overall health either. You can be overweight or obese and have normal blood test results and perfect blood pressure. It's just a shorthand that medical practitioners use to group patients into different categories of weight. This is what it looks like:

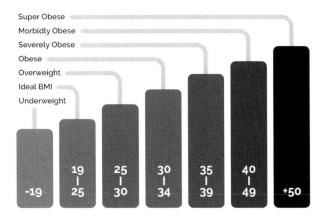

STANDARD MEDICAL BMI CHART

I think that the language in the commonly found chart above can be confusing—who decided that "super obese" is more obese than "severely obese"? I also don't like that they lump everyone in the 50+ BMI range into one category. In terms of disease progression and weight-loss success outcome statistics, someone at a 51 BMI is very different from someone at 100 BMI. While I am not a medical professional, I am going to take the liberty of creating my own chart and corresponding terms, ones that have a little less sticker shock and are, in my mind, a little more precise.

CUT GUT BMI CHART

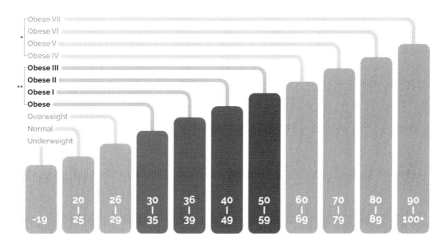

*People in the Obese IV–Obese VII categories have historically been the primary bariatric surgery patients.

**A shift is underway, and more people in the Obese–Obese III categories are discovering that they are excellent bariatric surgery candidates.

The Centers for Disease Control and Prevention (CDC) has found that the lowest mortality rates are among people whose body mass (according to the above chart) are in the normal and slightly overweight categories. This means that if you have a BMI near 25, you generally have the lowest chance of dying in your age group (notwithstanding other extenuating factors of course). Once you hit a BMI of 30, your chance of dying goes up precipitously as your BMI increases, due to comorbid conditions such as cardiovascular disease, type 2 diabetes, certain types of cancer, respiratory conditions like asthma and sleep apnea, and additional metabolic disorders.

It is worth noting that a long-held popular belief in the medical world seems to be that "thinner is healthier." This is not necessarily true. Katherine Flegal, an epidemiologist with the CDC, has found that the highest death rates are among those at either end of the BMI spectrum, and the lowest rates are in the normal BMI category. From a mortality perspective, extremely thin is not any healthier than extremely fat.

Being thin is also not morally superior. For those of you reading this who have never had a weight problem, I have an important message: *Many obese people are no different from you in terms of motivation, diet, exercise, and willpower.* At 123 pounds, I was eating greens and sweating to the oldies, and I was doing the same at my prewedding weight of 167 pounds. My first pregnancy took me to 220 pounds, but after my baby was born, I returned to 170 pounds; I wasn't so lucky after my second child, who arrived seven years later. I gained—and retained—68 pounds during that pregnancy, tipping the scales at 238 pounds after he was born, my highest set point to date. After his birth, I continued working out and eating healthfully, but the weight barely budged. I managed to fulfill my duties of a full-time partner, mother, and executive, all while killing myself trying to get thin, always chasing the next magic bullet.

Given that I spent so much of my life obsessing over health and body image, it may be hard to understand how there were periods of time that I seemed to lose track of my weight, or more accurately, I didn't seem to have a firm grasp on just how heavy I was getting. Unless you are fortunate enough to be one of those people who generally maintains a healthy weight within 5 to 10 pounds, it can be challenging for Looscy Larrys and Flying Fredas to keep consistent track of the Wonkavator rides their bodies like to take them on. If I wasn't vigorously dieting and constantly weighing myself, I became aware of my weight through happenstance, like seeing a random picture taken at a family gathering where I seemed to have suddenly developed a couple extra chins, or by seeing my reflection while walking by a glass high-rise window. *Do I really look like that?* I'd think. *That must be some fun-house mirror glass.*

Despite packing on the extra pounds, I *behaved* like a thin person, or at least how I'd been told a thin person behaved: counting every calorie, running miles and miles, and eating forests of kale. Some of the time—usually when I wasn't dieting—I felt I was only slightly overweight, even though I wasn't. Yes, it's true—sometimes denial kicked in. In my mind, I saw myself the way Hal saw Rosemary in the 2001 rom-com *Shallow Hal*. The movie's premise is that Rosemary, a fat woman, is gross and unlovable, and Hal needs to be hypnotized into seeing her "inner beauty," which of course looks exactly like a very thin Gwyneth Paltrow. Because I had once been thin, that's how I frequently saw myself: a thin girl in a fat girl's body. I'd be surprised when I went to the department store and found that the best fit was a size 20. After all that sweat and starvation, how could it be possible that I wasn't a size 8? I'd leave the dressing room deflated, the cycle of self-loathing would restart, and my weight and health obsession would return.

CHAPTER 2

They Want Their Cut

Stop looking for happiness in the
same place you lost it.
—Unknown

Let's say being 8 pounds above your ideal weight is analogous to having a scratch on your leg. It stings a bit, but it's relatively superficial. Being 22 pounds above your ideal weight is like having a small gash. It hurts more, and it goes deeper. Being 150 pounds above your ideal weight is like having part of your leg cut open, a big gaping wound that hurts like hell and potentially poses some serious health problems if it's not treated properly. Being 500 pounds over your ideal weight is like having your femoral artery cut through. Blood is spurting out like crazy, people are screaming, your vision is starting to go dark, and a light is appearing in the distance. There's a very good chance that you could *die*. OK, I know I'm getting a bit gory here, but stay with me for a minute. Out of these four injuries, in which would you apply a Band-Aid as the sole treatment? The scratch of course. It would work well too. But try putting one of those little beige bandages on a real gash, a deep cut, or an open femoral artery, and you'll have a big problem—and a bloody mess.

So why is it that almost every diet plan is the same whether you need to lose 8, 22, 150, or 500 pounds? Quitting alcohol and avoiding carbs after noon might work for someone with a bit of jiggle around their middle, but not so much for someone with type 2 diabetes and an extra 150 pounds on their frame. Let's face it: most diets are really meant for people who already have a normal BMI, those who want to lose 10 pounds before their wedding or drop a dress size before their twenty-year high school reunion.

Diets are a Band-Aid, an appropriate remedy for a superficial scratch but not really helpful for a deeper issue. And just as you can't wear a Band-Aid forever, a diet—rather than just plain old "healthy eating"—implies a beginning and an end. Consider the grapefruit diet that, according to WebMD, has been around since the 1930s. In this plan, you eat, drink, or take a pill containing grapefruit at every meal, cut way back on carbs, and increase your animal protein intake. According to certain proponents of the diet, grapefruit has some magical enzyme that burns fat. But in a randomized 2006 study from the Division of Endocrinology, Department of Nutrition and Metabolic Research, at Scripps Clinic in La Jolla, California, Dr. Kathleen Zelman clearly states that "grapefruit doesn't burn fat." The study did, however, demonstrate statistically significant weight loss (between 1.1 and 1.6 kilogram, or 2.4 to 3.5 pounds) in obese patients who took a grapefruit capsule, drank a glass of grapefruit juice, or ate a half grapefruit before each meal compared to those who took a placebo (0.3 gram). The study also found there was a reduction of two-hour post-glucose insulin levels in the grapefruit group. The sample size was small, with only ninety-one patients, and lasted only twelve weeks, so who knows if everyone was able to eat a grapefruit derivative three times a day for the rest of their lives, or if they gained the weight they lost after it ended. And it's unclear of what besides grapefruit the study's three daily meals consisted. Were participants indulging in BLTs and big bowls of fettuccine Alfredo, or were they eating spinach salads and half portions of vegan risotto?

Most variations of the grapefruit diet are essentially starvation diets, so in that way it does work, at least in the short term. When I was on it, I got down to approximately 1,000 calories a day. That's about half the recommended daily calorie intake for the average adult. But while eating fewer calories can help you lose weight, doctors generally don't endorse falling too far below your recommended daily intake. Doing so can cause symptoms like fatigue, constipation, light-headedness, and blurred vision. I vividly remember walking around the supermarket in a low-blood-sugar daze while I was on the grapefruit diet, sluggishly packing my shopping cart full of grapefruits. Eating too few calories when your metabolic feedback mechanisms are broken will likely sabotage your weight loss.

Health problems aside, another question is, how long can you sustain eating plans like the grapefruit diet? Can you imagine eating a low-calorie diet with a grapefruit or grapefruit juice at every meal every day for the rest of your life? It isn't terribly realistic. Even those diets that don't push calorie counting have their own limitations, and the claimed health benefits are, on the whole, unproven.

Boston Medical Center reported that of the estimated forty-five million Americans who go on an annual diet, 50 percent of them use fad diets. Fad diets go in and out of style because they generally promise dramatic weight-loss results via a level of calorie restriction that is unsustainable. They also frequently involve unhealthy, unbalanced eating plans that restrict entire food groups. "Fat free" was all the rage in the 1980s and 1990s, during which a whole bunch of processed and flavorless fat-free and low-fat products entered the market. Remember those fat-free Wow! chips with the fat-substitute olestra and the disclaimer "may cause abdominal cramping and loose stools" on the bag? No wonder those weren't around for very long.

Now, we understand that eating low fat doesn't always lead to losing fat, and the pendulum has swung in the other direction. Eating plans such as the paleo diet and ketogenic diet are all the rage. These diets are predicated on what we supposedly did when we were cavemen. There are several problems with building a modern lifestyle around an imagined past. Hunter-gatherers might have been mean and lean, but they were probably often malnourished and had all kinds of unfortunate diseases. Just because they ate wild, seasonal nuts and fruits (which would not be allowed or greatly minimized on a ketogenic diet anyhow) and ran in fast bursts every now and then doesn't necessarily mean they were healthier, at least not by today's standards. What with all those saber-toothed tigers running around and not a drop of penicillin to be had, the majority of these tribes didn't live too far past the age of thirty. Today, in the US, we live to an average of seventy-eight years old. It's impossible to compare our modern lifestyle to hunting and gathering on the African savanna.

How does eating processed food products like extra virgin coconut oil and low-carb almond-flour pizza crust or out-of-season South American–grown raspberries fit into this fantasy? Ancient wild game is not the same as the modern farm-raised cows, pigs, and chickens most of us have access to. If we're trying to emulate cavemen, should we really be eating out-of-season vegetables or antibiotic-laced foods, not to mention sodium-laden, processed low-carb bars, shakes, "treats," prepackaged meal kits, and frozen entrées?

Then there are the ethical and environmental implications of a high-meat diet. Scientists are encouraging all of us to drastically reduce our intake of animal protein to help sustain the planet, given the Earth's growing population and cascading ecological disasters. Because what's the point of being skinny if you have to live on a dying husk of a planet?

Let's examine these diets a little further. A primary difference between the paleo diet and the ketogenic diet is that people following the paleo diet get most of their calories from protein, whereas ketogenic dieters get most of their calories from fat. One key component of the paleo diet is to avoid grains, including whole grains. Although there is no clear scientific data to support it, paleo proponents claim that grains cause inflammation that can lead to an array of diseases and early death. For people with celiac disease like me (diagnosed in my early forties, years after all those nights at the pizza joint in college), certain whole grains do cause problems (such as damage to the small intestines). But for the other 98 percent of the population, is it really necessary to abolish an entire food group? According to Kelly Leveque, author of *Body Love: Live in Balance, Weigh What You Want, and Free Yourself from Food Drama Forever*, healthy carbohydrates contain important vitamins, minerals, and phytonutrients that help produce the mucus that protects our intestines and gut health. Besides, the energy created by healthy carbs is responsible for pretty much all of the best things in our modern world. The invention of agriculture allowed us to create food surplus, giving us the time and energy to devote to new and important endeavors, such as math, metalwork, indoor plumbing, the Sistine Chapel, and *The White Album*. Thank you, quinoa!

To better understand the argument *against* cutting out grains, we have to first understand that all grains contain three parts: the bran, the germ, and the endosperm. Whole grains use all three parts of the grain and are nutritionally superior to refined grains, which use only the endosperm. A 2007 Nurses' Health Study (NHS) of approximately 161,000 women focused on the possible risk of developing type 2 diabetes from a dietary intake of whole grains and bran. Women with the highest intake of whole grains were nearly 40 percent *less* likely to develop type 2 diabetes compared to women in the lowest intake group. While we've known for some time from the NHS study (and multiple other studies with similar findings) that whole grain intake actually reduces the rise of type 2 diabetes and cardiovascular disease, less was known about whole grain intake's correlation to death rates. So a major study was completed and published in *JAMA Internal Medicine* in which approximately 118,000 men and women were studied over a twenty-five-year period. In subjects who had the highest whole grain intake, there was a statistically significant (nearly 10 percent) reduction in death from all causes and a 15 percent reduction in cardiovascular disease–related death. The assertion that "all grains are bad" just doesn't hold up scientifically. It also seems that the paleo diet is different depending on whom you ask or which book you read, which can be very confusing. But not all aspects of the diet are bad. The paleo diet restricts processed foods and sugars and encourages exercise.

Similarly, the keto diet seeks to nearly eliminate carbohydrate intake (to only about 10 percent of your daily calories) while 60–80 percent of your calorie intake should be from fat, with the rest coming in the form of protein, all in an effort to put and keep a person's body in ketosis. Nutritional ketosis (rather than diabetic ketoacidosis, which is a life-threatening emergency) is when the body burns stored fat through ketones for energy instead of glucose/blood sugar. While I have the same fundamental concerns with the near total elimination of entire food groups (some parts of those food groups containing healthy whole foods), this diet trains the brain and allows it to run mutually exclusive energy sourcing from carbohydrates via glucose or fats via ketones, which is not a bad thing. Think of your brain as a hybrid car, able to burn energy from two kinds of energy sources (gasoline/glucose and electricity/ketones) rather than being solely dependent on just one energy source. Between 2008 and 2016, Florida neonatologist Dr. Mary T. Newport performed some interesting experiments with her husband Steve, using ketones as an alternative fuel for the brain—not for weight loss but toward the continuing quest to find a cure for Alzheimer's. I am not saying there is not a place for a ketogenic diet, particularly when, for some, genetic or environmental health factors might cause the benefits to outweigh the possible risks (such as high cholesterol from too much fat intake). However, the average healthy adult continuously rejecting glucose as a source of energy (via fresh whole berries, organic whole grains, sweet potatoes, and chickpeas) seems unnecessary, not to mention nearly impossible to sustain long term.

This brings me to the vegan diet. I think we can all agree that this has a leg up on the morality front, since animals and their by-products aren't being farmed, using up valuable environmental resources. Also, we are not killing other creatures for human consumption. But is a vegan diet sustainable? For some, yes, such as the guy my family met in Hawaii who is a proud vegan, sells kombucha, lives in a comfortable vitamin D–rich climate, and eats local plants widely available and rich in macro- and micronutrients. For me—and for many others—not so much. After a few months on a vegan diet, I started to have trouble sleeping and staying focused. And I started craving cheese with the kind of fervor that kept me up at night. Every now and then I'd sleep-walk, coming to in front of my refrigerator, staring at my empty cheese tray. So that didn't last long.

With a few exceptions, no diet can be a forever diet. Healthy eating is one thing; cutting out all foods from a certain group or drastically restricting calories is another. Have you ever vowed to stay on a par-ticular diet for life? If so, have you succeeded? My guess is no, which is why you are reading this book. It's not really possible for most of us to live on juice indefinitely, or to resist carbohydrates for the rest of our days. To do so requires the type of vigilance that makes real life—not to mention genuine pleasure—next to impossible. I've known people who are so focused on maintaining their diet that they give up living life; in fact, I've been one of them. And I can tell you that it's a miser-able way to live.

Can't Cut the Mustard

The Biggest Loser, the weight-loss reality TV show that ran for seven-teen seasons between 2004 and 2016 and inspired a plethora of inter-national spin-offs, showed the world just how unsustainable extreme dieting is. Reality TV is by its very nature extreme: the young women on *The Bachelor* backstab and seduce to win a husband; groups of strangers jump off cliffs to survive on *Survivor*; and the mixed martial arts fighters kick each other in the face to win contracts with the UFC on *The Ultimate Fighter*. (Really, the only civilized competitive reality show is *The Great British Baking Show*.) As in most reality TV shows, *The Biggest Loser* contestants did extraordinary and at times ludicrous things to achieve their goals.

Every *The Biggest Loser* season opened with the dreaded weigh-in, in which each contestant faced the scale in front of their team, their competitors, and all of America. Tears were shed, shame was spread. After every segment on the show—from the personal training sessions to the sadistic "temptation," in which contestants had to decide whether they would eat a piece of chocolate cake or stay on the diet and receive a gift, such as a phone call home—everyone got weighed. Then the team of the person who lost the least amount of weight had to vote someone off the show.

I was a huge fan of *The Biggest Loser*. I cheered on my fellow weight warriors, season after season. I shed many tears and sweat right along with them, from the comfort of my couch. I admired them. I knew their struggles all too well. I felt their pain, deeply. I related to these people, identified with them—they were *me*! If they could do it, so could I. Each week I'd watch with bated breath as they stepped onto the scale. I cried with them, laughed with them, and rooted for them. I wanted each and every fat person on that show to *win*.

Apparently, only one of the couples that emerged out of twenty-two seasons of *The Bachelor* is still together. Does this surprise you? It's hard enough for regular people leading regular lives to hold on to a relationship; it's all but impossible for a romance forged in such a contrived setting to survive in the real world. The same goes for weight loss: a major drop on the scale in such an artificial environment cannot survive in the real world. Unfortunately, most of *The Biggest Loser* contestants have regained much (if not all) of the weight they so arduously lost. In fact, a 2016 study published in *Scientific American* found that, out of fourteen contestants and study participants on season 8, thirteen had gained the weight back, and four of those thirteen were heavier than they had been before the competition.

You can go online to find reports of how the show's extreme diet tactics may have permanently damaged the contestants' metabolisms, and articles about many contestants' almost Herculean efforts to keep the weight off once the show was over. Still, I've seen comments from disappointed viewers saying that the contestants had "won the lottery" by getting to be on the show and then just let old habits creep back in again. That's straight-up rude. More importantly, it's wrong.

We should all thank *The Biggest Loser* for giving the contestants a venue for showing the world how deeply committed so many obese people are to losing weight. The contestants on the show were willing to put themselves in extreme situations and at great cost. They had a ton of chutzpah! These clearly determined people should be thanked for their gift to science. Through their grit and hard work, they demonstrated just how difficult it is for fat people to lose weight and keep it off, no matter how hard we work. Now we can quit playing the blame game and focus our attention on finding solutions to the underlying problem of metabolic disease.

Of course, *The Biggest Loser* is not the main culprit here. The show is just a symptom of the problem, a microcosm of what's wrong with the way our society approaches weight loss. Somehow, we've all come to share the delusion that extreme dieting and exercise work, even though there is no real evidence to back up the claim. A healthy diet and regular exercise keep already fit people fit. Diets work best for people who really don't need to diet in the first place. So why do we stubbornly continue to apply that same formula to people who have been obese for ten years or more?

Director's Cut

In order to complete my master's of education in Human Resources, Occupational Training, and Development and Instructional Design (a fancy way of saying "teaching, primarily in a business setting"), I was required to provide a certain number of training hours to test subjects. They were volunteers, mostly poor college students like myself, to whom I had to teach a variety of random things, from quantum physics to how to make a peanut-butter-and-jelly sandwich. While I taught, each test subject was hooked up to electrodes that monitored their brain activity, and their brains had to light up in a certain way in order for the training to be deemed effective. In other words, the test subjects had to learn something.

During the first training I conducted, no one lit up. I was an abject failure. Apparently, those damn people weren't paying attention! What a bunch of flakes. Or maybe they were just plain stupid. Or hungover—they were college students, after all. Whatever it was, I had no doubt that they were to blame.

My professor did not agree. Much to my chagrin, he sat me down afterward and asked me what I thought I had done wrong.

"What do you mean, what did *I* do wrong?" I asked. "*They're* the students. It was their responsibility to perform."

"If people do not learn in your class," the professor said pointedly, "it is your responsibility."

Before that moment, I'd believed that if I didn't do well in school, it was my fault. If I failed an exam, it was because I hadn't studied hard enough. If I didn't get an A on a paper, it was because I hadn't worked hard enough. If I didn't understand a concept, it was because I hadn't thought hard enough. Blaming the teacher was never an option. This is what my family and childhood community had taught me, intentionally or not.

"And if they don't pass, you won't graduate," my teacher added.

"That's just not fair," I said.

"Each person who signed up for these training sessions expressed a full willingness to learn. That was part of the deal. And whatever's standing in their way, it's your job to help them overcome it."

This conversation rattled me. It was true that the students had given me their undivided attention, and they seemed to truly be engaged. Then there was the fact that they had submitted themselves to the experiment in the first place, to wearing electrodes on their heads for a couple hours at a time. Would they really go to all that trouble to simply slack off in the end?

Slowly, I came to accept that the students' willingness to learn was the most that I could ask for. My job—my duty—was to keep their attention by whatever means necessary, to create an instructional design full of eye-catching visuals, colorful examples, and captivating dialogue. I had to stop blaming the students and become the kind of teacher that inspires and enables learning.

Once my attitude changed, so did my curriculum and facilitation. I'd been humbled, an essential part of any good education. I began to recognize the students' blank stares, and instead of passing over them in disgust, I changed my instructional direction when I noticed them. I became more empathetic, another education essential. Most important, I no longer viewed their failure to learn as their fault; instead, I knew if they were willing and able but still failing, it was my shortcoming.

Where am I going with all this? You guessed it: this is another allegory for dieting, in which the students represent the obese dieters, and I play the role of the diet industry. What if fat people weren't to blame, but instead the fault lay with the diet industry? What if we stopped beating fat people over the head with old dieting methodology dressed up with a new name? What if we accepted that dieting just doesn't work for *most* people with long-term 30+ body mass index (BMI)?

The thing is, weight-loss companies have to claim that their diets work for everyone. That's why the promises are oblique and their oversized claims always come with fine print. If you take a few minutes to peruse the diet interwebs, it'll become clear early on that for every evidence-based claim that the sky is blue, there is an equally convincing claim that the sky is a robust plaid. For those of us who are not statisticians, data analysts, or economists, it can be difficult and frustrating to try to separate the wheat from the chaff, the fact from the fiction.

It might take you a while to find it, but it is worth your time to read the fine print. One diet recommends eating lean protein, "heart-healthy" fat, and "good" carbs to "transform" your metabolism, and its specialty products can be delivered to your door. At the time of this writing, the homepage on its website says, "Lose up to 7 lbs. in your first 7 days." You'll notice that it says nothing about keeping that weight off (and for someone who's morbidly obese, 7 pounds matters, but it's also little more than a drop in the bucket). There's an asterisk (there's always an asterisk) that points to more information written in a teeny-weeny font that states that, in the four-week study this claim is based on, the average weight loss was 5.8 pounds in the first seven days, not the 7 pounds claimed in big letters above. If you click on the link, you'll see some not-so-promising language that reads, "Many commer cial products/diet plans are readily available to the weight-conscious consumer; however, evidence specific to their tolerance and weight-loss promoting effectiveness is often lacking." Click on the "Success Stories" link, and you'll find a bunch of "before" and "after" photos. From my vantage point, the people in the photos look like a bunch of normal-weight people who went from having a little softness at the waistline to six-pack abs.

The same goes for another popular weight-loss program that's promoted online. If "Lose All the Weight You Want for $49 (plus the cost of food)" sounds too good to be true, that's because it is. The company website claims that "successful weight loss and weight management can be achieved through a healthy relationship with food, an active lifestyle, and a balanced approach to living." That's not *not* true, but it isn't very specific. The copy on the site is written in a kind of code: "[Our] tools, along with our more than 600 brick and mortar centers, help our potential members take immediate and lasting advantage of what we call 'The I'm ready to lose weight NOW' moment." What the hell does that mean? Such vague language pro-tects the company from litigation. Imagine a plaintiff trying to prove that a diet company didn't help him take advantage of his "I'm ready to lose weight NOW" moment!

You have to root around the website for a while for anything that clarifies the company's vague weight-loss claims. Again, there's the big writing: "Lose up to 16 pounds in your first 4 weeks," and then the asterisk: "Avg. weight loss in studies was 11.6 lbs. for those who completed the program." Click on the link, and you'll discover that the study participants ate 1,200 to 2,000 calories' worth of this company's brand breakfast, lunch, dinner, snack, and bars or shakes per day and attended five weekly consultations for a full four weeks. Five sessions per week! Who's got the time for that?

And another company's big print: "Lose up to 13 lbs. & 7 inches overall in your first month!" Asterisk: "Avg. weight loss in study was 11.6 lbs. and 8 inches." Click on the link: the study is only four weeks, and participants are on what is essentially a starvation diet, eating between 1,000 and 1,500 calories per day. (Maybe someone from the marketing department should update their "inches lost" claim. The actual averages apparently outperformed the advertised amount!)

I could go on, and on, and on.

Anyway, we could starve ourselves for free! So why do we spend almost $70 billion and counting every year on diets? Because the industry is a vast machine that preys on the two most powerful of human emotions: shame and hope. Diet companies spend hundreds of millions of dollars on disingenuous ad campaigns that spread the cultural message that fatness is badness, and then offer a solution that, if you read the fine print, is no solution at all. Mostly, these campaigns are designed to make fat people feel ashamed (though they'd never cop to this agenda) and keep us coming back for more of the same. Shame keeps us quiet, secretive, and all too easy to manipulate. Hope makes millions of Americans dream of a better, thinner tomorrow. Hope makes us keep our skinny wardrobe at the back of our closets, behind the clothing that actually fits. Hope makes us tell ourselves, *I'll lose 50 pounds by summer*, then amend it to autumn, then winter, and then the year 2030. Hope convinces us that, even though the past two hundred diets we tried didn't work, somehow diet number 201 is going to be the ticket to significant and sustainable weight loss. When it doesn't work, shame replaces hope. And the cycle continues.

Now, I'm not saying that there's some evil puppet master pulling at our heartstrings. There are plenty of well-intentioned weight-loss companies run by people who truly believe in what they are peddling. But there are also plenty of others just looking for a way to turn a profit with a product or service that they know is the same old zebra with slightly different stripes.

Cut a Check

So how does the diet industry keep us coming back again and again and again? Why do we get selective amnesia when a coworker mentions this *amazing* new diet that we just *have to* try? I believe that celebrities play a big part. They're talented, beautiful, and rich—everything we're supposed to aspire to be. Plus, if they have an apparent weight-loss success story, we forget there's a reason they made it onto our screens in the first place: namely, their power to sell an image. And they're usually being paid handsomely for that power.

The next time you're admiring a gorgeous, recently slimmed-down actress in your news feed, give yourself a pinch and a reality check. You think Jessica Simpson, Jennifer Hudson, and Marie Osmond lost 50 or 80 pounds through moderate exercise and sticking to the meal plan? Maybe. Perhaps they had somehow missed the memo about healthy diet and regular exercise, and then, when a diet company shared the good news, all they had to do was switch out jelly beans for broccoli and they were off and running. That's not how it works for most of us, and I think it's safe to assume that it probably doesn't work that way for the rich and famous either.

Some dieters truly can lose 100 pounds and keep it off through diet and exercise, but they are the rare exception. Celebrities are such successful weight-loss spokespeople in part because they can pay professionals to make them look good, to give them perfect hair, a flawless pedicure, and just the right lighting. They can afford to hire personal trainers, massage therapists, acupuncturists, hypnotherapists, and Le Cordon Bleu–trained chefs who manage to turn a sliver of salmon, a sprig of dill, and five capers into a glorious feast. Add to that the best girdle money can buy and an expert makeup artist, and you've got an hourglass figure and icepick cheekbones. And if all else fails, there are a plethora of plastic surgeons who would be happy to help. Celebrities can treat thinness as a full-time job because, for most of them, it's an essential job requirement in our fat-shaming culture.

It goes without saying that most of us can't work the full-time weight-loss job necessary to subvert nature. Most of us are busy working our actual full-time jobs. Then there's folding the laundry, washing the dishes, mowing the lawn, walking the dog, and making sure little Jimmy is doing his homework, all of which takes priority over climbing those extra two miles on the StairMaster. We have lives to live.

And even with all the resources and support in the world, celebrities often gain the weight back. Oprah, whose stake in Weight Watchers is estimated to be worth hundreds of millions, is famous for her weight yo-yoing over the years. Kirstie Alley lost her Jenny Craig contract after gaining back some of the 75 pounds she'd dropped. In 2014, she got back on the wagon and re-signed. In a *People* article from that year, she says something that breaks my heart. "Like I say in the ad, I'm not circus fat. I didn't hugely screw up. I didn't gain 75. I gained 30." I can't believe they green-lighted the phrase "circus fat" in 2014!

I'm not a big fan of celebs' "before and after" and "after-the-after photos." Those photos don't tell us their resting heart rate or blood pressure, how good they feel, or how personally fulfilled they are. We don't know if those high cheekbones indicate a joyful life or one consumed by hunger and misery. Plus, these photos reinforce our impulse to make judgments based on appearances, particularly on women's appearances (you'll notice that most weight-loss spokespeople are women).

The sad truth is that when a weight-loss spokesperson gains weight, the harsh light of public blame is all too quick to bear down upon them. In a 2011 *New York Times* article, Zalmi Duchman, the chief executive of Fresh Diet, didn't hesitate to throw the company's spokesperson under the bus. "If they don't do good on it, it doesn't mean the product doesn't work," he said. "It just means that they're not sticking to it." We immediately assign blame to the dieter, and we revel in those gossip mags that show zoomed-in photos of actresses' upper-thigh cellulite, post-baby potbellies, and soft under-chins. I've bought those rags to feel a warped kind of comfort, to relish celebrities' public shaming while keeping my own shame private. Pointing fingers is easy;

it's harder to empathize and investigate, to pause for a moment and question why so many dieters—even the rich and famous ones—can't keep the weight off.

Cut from the Same Cloth

There's an old joke, which goes something like this:

A guy goes to see his doctor. "Doc," he says, "you got to help me."

"What seems to be the matter?" the doctor asks.

"I get terrible headaches."

The doctor lists off the possible causes. Dehydration? No. Too much screen time? Nope. Stress levels? No more than average. Too much booze? Nah. Finally, after exhausting the usual suspects, the doctor says, "Well, let's run some tests."

The patient goes through every evaluation and test known to man. Everything comes back negative. Discouraged, the doctor says, "I don't know what to tell you. Is there anything you can think of, anything you forgot to tell me?"

"Oh, yeah," the man says. "I forgot to mention one thing. It usually starts to hurt every time I do this." He then proceeds to slam his head into the wall.

That was me and dieting. I've said it before and I'll say it again: I've tried everything. Atkins, paleo, ketogenic, and veganism. Gluten free. The grapefruit diet. The South Beach Diet. Weight Watchers, Jenny Craig, Nutrisystem, Optifast, and many, many more. For me, following each diet was like slamming my head against the wall. I would commit heart and soul to a prescribed plan and sometimes didn't lose anything more than a pound or two. Other times, I'd lose a significant number of pounds at the offset, up to 25 percent of my excess weight. Euphoria would ensue. I'd found it, the cure to my obesity! It would be smooth sailing from here on out. Then my body would adapt to the calorie deprivation or the state of ketosis and I'd hit a plateau. Even if I continued to cling to the regime by the skin of my teeth (while both daydreaming and night-dreaming about all the food I was denying myself), the weight I lost would creep back up. Imagine what it feels like to be standing on the scale after two months of torturous calorie restriction and, your belly rumbling, see that you've actually gained weight since you started the diet! I'll tell you what it feels like: slamming your head against a wall.

But I kept chasing the dream. I craved the elation I'd experience when I lost significant weight at the start of some diets, a sensation that was the opposite of a head slam. Nothing in this world feels better than putting on a pair of jeans to find that they aren't as tight as they were last week. Those little moments of happiness keep us coming back for more, like bad boy (or girl) types who kiss like a dream but never call us back. Some of us just keep going, hoping that if we do everything right, maybe this one will be the One.

I call those of us in this category Fluffins. If you are a Fluffin, some or all of the below statements will ring true:

- You are a disciplined person. You work hard and are successful in many aspects of your life, from your career and finances to your personal relationships.
- You are nearly 100 percent compliant when you are on a diet. You do not "closet" (secretly) eat, and you don't succumb to "cheat days" when you feel like quitting.
- Your skinny/normal weight friends and family seem to eat more than you do, and they can't understand why you are overweight.
- You are active and exercise regularly.
- You have tried many diet-and-exercise plans over the last decade with the following results: you lose 20 percent or

less of your extra weight and gain it right back when you stop the diet. Or on the rare occasions that you have lost a significant amount of weight, you gain all or most of it back within one year.

- The famous line "Insanity is doing the same thing over and over again and expecting different results" (misattributed to Albert Einstein, original source unknown) frequently plays in your head.

- You feel hopeless and frustrated because you have tried everything and yet still cannot achieve and/or maintain significant weight loss. You have recurring thoughts that go something like *Why am I so fluffy? I should be* thin *based on the number of diets I've tried, my general lifestyle, and activity level.*

If you haven't peed on a stick to check whether you are in ketosis in the last couple years, if you don't know that 5:2 is not just an answer on your seventh-grader's math homework, and if you haven't had a workout so grueling that you threw up, chances are you are not a Fluffin.

Instead, you might be more like my friend Anthony. At 6 feet 5 and around 350 pounds, he's a big, happy bear of a man. His pride and joy is his twenty thousand dollars' worth of barbeque equipment, on which he makes the most succulent, mouthwatering ribs you'll ever eat. He loves food, unabashedly and unapologetically. He also has a sense of humor about his weight. "I'm going to have a heart attack!" he'll joke over a plate of sauce-drenched flank steak.

As one fat person to another, I've been comfortable sharing my own weight struggles with him over the years. "I lost X pounds on my new diet!" I've told him proudly many times. Then, a couple weeks later, I've reported sadly, "I gained X + 3 pounds." He'd nod his head and give me a reassuring pat on the back. He'd been through that wringer before, with the same unsatisfactory results, and he knew the emotional ups and downs that come with weight loss and gain. More recently, he's admitted to me that he's been diagnosed as prediabetic and that he truly does worry about having a heart attack before his kids are grown. "But," he's said, "why bother killing myself for nothing? I'd do something about my weight if it worked. Until a real solution comes along, I'm just going to enjoy my life while I can."

Anthony is what I call a DietDisser. He has decided that enough is enough. If you have too, some or all of the below statements will ring true:

- You have the discipline to follow a diet, but you aren't giving in to all of the hype. You enjoy food and drink, and you are not going to stand on your head and eat grapefruit four times a day just because it's the latest craze and everyone else is doing it.
- You have watched your colleague limp around the office after throwing out his back doing a "workout of the day" (WOD) at the local CrossFit and secretly thought, *What an idiot!*
- You've "been there, done that" too many times to count, with little to no positive impact on your weight. Now you have consciously or unconsciously decided to live life as you are (at least for right now).
- You believe it is a wise decision not to push your body too hard through dieting, but you also don't feel very good. You have daily or hourly thoughts like *How much longer am I going to live? How am I going to face my family as I develop illnesses due to weight-related conditions?*

If you are a DietDisser, then congratulations: you called bullshit long before I did! But whether you are a DietDisser or a Fluffin, or a special snowflake (i.e., nobody's putting a label on me) and one of the millions of people struggling with long-term obesity, this book is for you. Let's stop slamming our heads against the wall and finally find a real solution to our nation's weight epidemic.

CHAPTER 3

Cut the Yayo

Talk about ya-yo, uhh, it's everywhere you go
They said in Miami, it'll never snow
Now it's snow in the palm trees, snow on the sand
It snows all day, for sixty dollars a gram
—Grandmaster Melle Mel

Katherine, one of my roommates in college, hit all the marks: smart, personable, and gorgeous. She was also bound by a strict religion that did not tolerate any drug use. But Katherine had struggles that eventually superseded her religious convictions. She felt she needed help maintaining the circumference of her upper thighs. She wanted "thigh gap," people! Katherine's aid of choice: cocaine. Her philosophy: if you can't tone it, TAN IT. If you can't drop it, POP IT (or snort it or shoot it).

In the short seven months that I lived with her, she did achieve that thigh gap. She also developed a well-hidden cocaine addiction that later led her to leaving school and seeking drug treatment. Sadly, she was disowned by her strictly religious family.

More recently, I worked with a guy in his midforties who told any-one who would listen that he'd had a severe weight problem for years but had found the solution. He was indeed thin, if a bit gaunt.

The guy's treatment of choice: a diet of alcohol. His philosophy: skip the calories (and money) spent on food and replace them with far fewer calories from alcohol (which also suppresses the appetite).

This gentleman was a self-proclaimed "drunkorexic." Drunkorexia is a growing phenomenon. Media about this disordered behavior tends to focus on college-aged people (mostly women), but its popularity is growing among adults in general, and one 2017 study found it affected men and women equally.

Katherine and the "alcohol as a primary caloric source" guy aren't the first people to use substances for weight loss, and I'd wager a guess that they won't be the last. We know their strategies are faulty, unhealthy, and not sustainable in the long run (and probably not so great for our personal relationships, families, or jobs either). The real question is, are there drugs (legal or otherwise) out there worth con-sidering for healthy, significant, and sustaining weight loss?

Cutting a Line

A central nervous system stimulant, amphetamine, was first synthe-sized in the late nineteenth century, but it wasn't until the 1920s that people began to see its pharmaceutical potential. This substance was first used as a decongestant in the form of an inhaler, and subsequent research and development found it to be useful for treating narcolepsy and depression. In fact, amphetamine was the first medication used as an antidepressant!

In 1929, chemist Gordon Alles had a colleague inject him with 50 milligrams of the stuff (back then, doctors experimenting on them-selves was a pretty common and accepted practice), and his nose cleared up like magic. His heart started to race, and he was filled with an expansive sense of well-being. He also felt smarter and more charismatic than usual—if only we had the input of his tablemates at the dinner party he attended that evening to verify, or contradict, his assertion about how witty he was. (If you've ever hung out with someone on speed, you know that while they might think they're entertaining, they're usually simply sped up and often annoying.) After the party, his heart rate decreased and he came down emotionally but had trouble sleeping.

Alles thought that, if amphetamine could work so well on sinus congestion, then perhaps it would help with asthma as well. (He had yet to seriously consider the ways it might be used to boost energy and mood.) Alles tested his treatment on patients suffering from asthma but found that it didn't do much for their wheezing. It did, however, give them that warm euphoric feeling, which was no small thing. After getting a US patent in 1932, Alles teamed up with the pharmaceutical firm Smith, Kline & French to explore how else amphetamines might be used.

Online you can find old black-and-white images of happy energetic people advertising Benzedrine sulfate tablets as prototypical antidepressants and mood elevators. *The Wizard of Oz* came out in 1939 and starred Judy Garland, who would die of a drug overdose years later at age forty-seven. Her own mother gave the seventeen-year-old uppers to make her performance as Dorothy more energetic. By the time World War II rolled around in the 1930s to 1940s, these amphetamine tablets—also known as "bennies"—were considered a credible psychiatric medication, and they'd become commercially successful across the country. The few reports of abuse that did emerge were ignored.

Not only did bennies seem to help alleviate depression; they also kept air force servicemen awake for the long flights into and out of war zones (and to take the edge off the sharp fact that, if you weren't shot out of the sky by enemy flak, you were likely to die due to a malfunction in one those janky airplanes). The US and British military supplied Benzedrine to their military while the Axis powers gave their soldiers a similar drug called Pervitin.

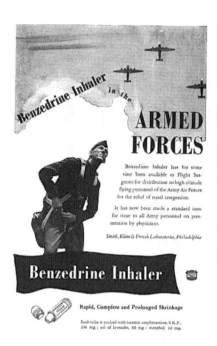

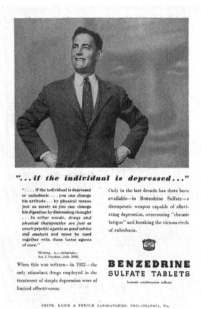

As American service people were fighting high overseas, classic film actors and directors, such as Marilyn Monroe, Mickey Rooney, and David O. Selznick, were using stimulants to work grueling hours. In fact, many Hollywood studios had their own doctors who freely prescribed the big names "pep pills" and "vitamin shots." The unknowns were using too; it is estimated that, by the end of the war, half a million American civilians were taking amphetamines at home.

The big added bonus of these pills: they kept people slim by speeding up the body's metabolic rate and suppressing appetite.

Dexedrine and Obetrol came onto the scene after the war. Some continued to use these substances for depression, some for weight loss, and some for all-night beatnik dance parties. Rumor has it that Jack Kerouac used meth in the late 1940s, and in the 1960s President John F. Kennedy received shots of methamphetamines from "Dr. Feelgood" to help him deal with Addison's disease as well as the pressures of the White House. At the same time, those old black-and-white ads started targeting depressed housewives and young coeds, showing smiling, apron-wearing white ladies happily vacuuming or smiling white ladies holding books, their berets jauntily askew. Another target demographic was "reducers," people who had fallen "victim to overeating and underactivity" who needed a little help ramping up their "stick-to-it-iveness."

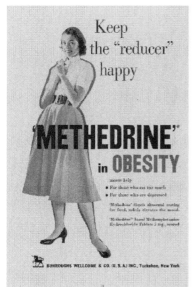
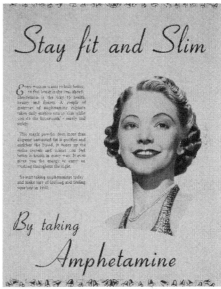

By 1962, American pharmaceutical companies were producing eighty thousand kilograms of amphetamine salts per year, the equivalent of forty-three standard 10-milligram doses *per person* in the US population at the time. In the United Kingdom, 3 percent of retail prescriptions filled in the Newcastle area were for amphetamines. About one-third were prescribed for depression or anxiety, one-third for nonspecific psychosomatic complaints like general tiredness, and one-third for weight loss.

Betty Friedan's 1963 bestseller, *The Feminine Mystique*, questioned the roots of white housewives' unhappiness. According to her, being perky, beautiful, and domestically efficient were not, in fact, women's most noble missions, despite advertisers' claims. Procuring the latest cleaning technology and attaining girlish slimness wasn't the solution to middle-class white female unrest, she argued. Perhaps some women, she said, wanted an education, work, or to have political opinions.

Cultural change was in the air throughout the United States and other parts of the globe. In the early 1970s, cardiologist Robert Atkins founded the Atkins diet. He believed that a high-protein, low-carb diet was more effective for long-term weight loss than drug-fueled starvation diets because, he argued, restricting carbohydrates forced your body to burn fat instead of carbs, and voilà, extra fat would melt away and stay off.

Meanwhile, the addictiveness of amphetamines was becoming clear. The drug was relatively easy to come by for pharma companies and even individual doctors, and could be subsequently sold for huge profits. Due to high accessibility and low oversight, many people had gotten hooked over the previous three decades. In 1970, it was determined that 970,000 amphetamine users in the United States met some criteria for dependence, and 320,000 could be considered addicts. And this is likely a conservative estimate.

Soon thereafter, the US government created the 1970 Comprehensive Drug Abuse Prevention and Control Act, and the Food and Drug Administration cracked down, making amphetamines a Schedule II drug. A Schedule II drug is a substance that has a "high potential for abuse" that could lead to "severe psychological or physical dependence," according to the US Drug Enforcement Administration (DEA). This regulation mostly included the more hard-core injectable products; more than six thousand oral amphetamine products were still considered Schedule III and in circulation on the US drug market. In 1971, all amphetamine products became Schedule II after it came to light that 80 to 90 percent of amphetamines confiscated on the street were manufactured by pharmaceutical companies. More rigorous standards of record keeping and distribution were set, and those companies were given strict production quotas. As the public lost access to amphetamines, cocaine and other street drugs filled the hole that they left in the market.

Gutsy Gal

Do you remember Anna Nicole Smith? She was a Guess Jeans girl and Playboy model who died way too young, in 2007 at the age of thirty-nine. I am fascinated by her story: an abusive childhood in the flatlands of Texas, a teenage pregnancy, minimum-wage work at Walmart and Red Lobster, a Marilyn Monroe–inspired makeover, and a career in stripping. She scrimped and saved for the DD breasts that allowed her to move up the stripping ladder to a fancier gentlemen's club, where she met the ninetysomething billionaire oil tycoon J. Howard Marshall whom she'd later marry. (Though she would be painted as the conniving gold digger, he pursued her for years before she finally agreed to marry him.) Hers is a real American Dream story in that she truly came from nothing and made a life for herself. Unfortunately, she's known best for her last years, during which the E! network recorded her sad decline.

The Anna Nicole Show ran from 2002 to 2004. Now something of a cult classic, it went off the air after three seasons and twenty-eight episodes due to poor ratings. After the show's cancellation, Smith became a spokesperson from 2004 to 2006 for a weight-loss drug. On YouTube, you can find an excruciating 2004 interview with Jay Leno, the kind that would no longer fly, at least not on mainstream late-night TV. In the episode, he *surveys the audience* about her then recent weight loss, asking them whether they think she should gain or lose any additional weight or if she looks OK as is. He then asks Smith about her sex life. He even encourages her to show off her lower-back tattoo to viewers. She appears to be game, fully embracing the ditzy blonde bombshell persona. That was how she earned a living, after all.

During the interview, Smith also blatantly promotes the weight-loss drug, claiming it had "shrunk" her stomach so she wasn't hungry, resulting in a loss of 69 pounds. All it took was six pills a day! During the two years of her ad campaign, the company's sales went up by 172 percent.

Anna Nicole Smith's story did not have a happy ending. Five months before she died, her own son lost his life to a drug overdose. When she died, she was on antibiotics for a massive infection throughout her body. It had developed from abscesses that had formed at injection sites where she'd received growth hormones. She was also on a number of substances, including Klonopin, Ativan, Valium, and the sleeping medication chloral hydrate. According to a bodyguard and other household staff, she washed these drugs down with copious amounts of expensive champagne and other alcoholic beverages.

Given everything she was on, it's hard to say what exactly caused all that weight loss. Certainly, she wasn't healthy. But the company used her celebrity to push a pill that, like many diet programs, drew upon a limited amount of data to substantiate its claims. And still, more than a decade after her death, Anna Nicole Smith is still featured prominently on the weight-loss drug's website.

Gut-Cutting Medications and Supplements

The social opinion, legality, and popularity of different drugs is always changing, and some people hurt themselves abusing the same drugs that others use to great benefit in moderation. Perhaps Anna Nicole Smith had some demons to outrun, and by all appearances she used substances for this purpose. Who can blame her? We all find ways to get high in our lives, whether it's through cold-water plunges or short-lived romances or yoga in 115-degree heat. Or stimulants.

The pursuit of euphoria is longstanding—even our hairier cousins indulge in it. In a 2001 report from the Primate Research Institute, Kyoto University found that apes not only take substances to fight against the parasites responsible for dysentery and malaria but also eat the seeds of Kola trees to get high off the caffeine and theobromine (yes, that's the same theobromine found in cacao, the main ingredient in chocolate). I doubt that our simian relatives use these drugs for weight management, but I can tell you that we humans often resort to substances to get high as well as to curb hunger, to make us feel fuller faster, or speed up metabolism. People in parts of Africa and the Arabian Peninsula chew the leaves and twigs of the East African evergreen shrub khat, or sprinkle it on food or turn it into tea in order to increase alertness and energy and reduce appetite (common side effects: cardiac complications, manic behavior with grandiose delusions, and insomnia). The tropical tree Kratom is native to Southeast Asia, and in small doses, consumption produces stimulant effects including appetite suppression. Peruvians chew coca leaves, which act as a mild stimulant, suppressing hunger, thirst, pain, and fatigue and helping them keep their energy up for long mountain treks in the Andes. During the 1980s fashion models snorted it to stay thin in its powdered form: cocaine. Because of its stimulant effect, coca leaf was originally used in the soft drink Coca Cola. In 1903 it was removed and a decocainized coca extract was used instead.

Like Benzedrine sulfate tablets and some other forms of amphetamines, these drugs happen to be banned by the Drug Enforcement Administration at the present moment, but uses and government sanctioning are always evolving, depending on what's new, what's in fashion, and who's in charge. Amphetamines happen to no longer be in style, at least not legally. But there's always something stimulating or appetite suppressing or that claims to aid weight reduction: nicotine, laxatives, caffeine, crack, diuretics, ephedrine, castor oil and mineral oil, Dr. Kellogg's infamous yogurt enemas, homeopathic pills, Epsom salts and milk of magnesia, energy drinks, dark chocolate, the flapper's diet of cigarettes and celery, and even arsenic, just to name a few—all of these have been used for weight loss at one time or another.

These days, there are about a million Library of Congresses' worth of weight-loss hacks, supplements, and herbal tricks online. Last week chili powder was the latest and greatest metabolism fixer; the week before, it was turmeric and aloe vera juice. A few years before that, coffee enemas were on trend. A decade before that, you could buy the stimulant ephedrine over the counter at health-and-fitness specialty stores. (Sad anecdote: The young wife of the owner of a company I used to work for took too much ephedrine, had a heart attack, and died. The drug has since been banned.)

You don't need a prescription for these supplements, many of which have "natural" ingredients like cinnamon, Garcinia cambogia, raspberry ketones, elephant yam fiber, mint, bitter orange, and other secret plant extracts. There is the tried-and-true stimulant caffeine in green tea extract and green coffee bean extract, as well as good ol' coffee and tea. Plus, we can always fall back on nicotine, which is highly effective in helping to suppress appetite, is highly addictive in its smoke form, causes cancer, and in its vaping form (in the United States) has suddenly, indiscriminately, and mysteriously killed multiple people!

As in monetized diet programs, scientific evidence for the long-term weight-loss efficacy of these substances is limited. Most supplement companies base their weight-loss claims on studies they themselves fund, and often these studies look at just a small sample size over the course of a few weeks. Some manufacturers use rats in their studies, and though we do have a lot in common, I think it's fair to say that there are enough differences between us that substances won't necessarily affect us the way they affect rodents.

More than that, most of their claims are simply not evaluated by the Food and Drug Administration. Maybe you trust the FDA, maybe you don't; but without any real oversight, it's a Wild West of over-the-counter weight-loss drugs, herbs, and supplements out there, with newfangled cure-alls hitting the market every day. And unless you have a lab in your basement and know how to use it, you really can't be sure what will harm and what will help.

Now, I'm not making a moral judgment on any of these medications, nor am I presuming to give health advice. I am not a doctor, and I fully respect each person's right to choose what they do with their body. I'd also bet that some of the weight-loss drugs and supplements I've discussed here have truly helped people to lose weight or address other health and wellness issues. That includes amphetamines: when prescribed appropriately and taken in carefully monitored doses, amphetamines can do a lot of good for people. I am a big fan of modern medicine and give full credit to prescription drugs for doing so much for humanity. (Imagine a world without penicillin, antibiotics, antihistamines, insulin, or antimalaria pills. And what if those British and American pilots hadn't done their jobs so well?)

You can still get a prescription for amphetamine derivatives if you set your mind to it. Variants of this stimulant are used in drugs for the treatment of attention deficit hyperactivity disorder (ADHD), the most well known being Adderall and Ritalin. Ritalin gained popularity in the early 1990s, along with some new weight-loss drugs, including fenfluramine-phentermine, commonly known as fen-phen. Fen-phen was abruptly banned from sale in 1997, when it was discovered to have a 20 percent risk of causing a lethal heart-valve injury for users. Other stimulant and amphetamine-derivative weight-loss drugs like Meridia, DMAA, and the supplement ephedra have come and gone, due to the risk they posed of causing cardiovascular problems, such as heart attack and stroke. Hundreds of reported cases of heart disease and a handful of deaths later, amphetamine-based diet drugs have become more heavily regulated and harder to come by.

As far as FDA-approved weight-loss drugs, there are still options, some with a low dosage of amphetamine, some without. Weight-loss pills are available by prescription and over the counter, and they use different mechanisms and come with different side effects. And no medical professionals are promising that any of these prescription pills are the sole key to weight loss. Lifestyle and diet are very much part of the prescription program. As it says on the National Institute of Diabetes and Digestive and Kidney Diseases website, medications don't replace physical activity or healthy eating habits.

In recent years, the FDA has approved five new drugs to combat obesity:

- **bupropion-naltrexone** (brand name: Contrave) is a combination antidepressant and smoking cessation aid (bupropion) and a medication that is also used to treat alcohol and opiod dependence (naltrexone), approved by the FDA in 2014. It works by lessening appetite and making you feel full faster.

> » Possible side effects include increased blood pressure, increased heart rate, headache, constipation, insomnia, nausea, vomiting, dry mouth, dizziness, diarrhea, liver damage, and suicidal ideation, among others.

- **liraglutide** (brand name: Saxenda) is an injection used for weight-loss and diabetes management, approved by the FDA in 2014. It works by lessening appetite and making you feel full faster.

  > » Possible side effects include nausea and vomiting, stomach pain, raised pulse, and headache, among others.

- **lorcaserin** (brand name: Belviq) is similar to fenfluramine but doesn't carry the same risk of damaging heart valves, approved by the FDA in 2012. It acts on the serotonin receptors in your brain and works by helping you feel full faster.

  > » Possible side effects include headache, nausea, back pain, dry mouth, dizziness, cough, and tiredness, among others. Patients are advised to avoid using with certain antidepressants or migraine medications.

- **orlistat** (brand name: Xenical) can be procured either as a prescription or in a reduced-strength over-the-counter form. It was approved by the FDA in 1999. This is the only weight-loss drug that is approved for children between the ages of twelve and eighteen. It works by reducing your body's absorption of fat, but you still have to maintain a low-fat diet.

> » Possible side effects include gastrointestinal complaints like increased flatulence, loose and oily stools, and stomach pain, among others.

- **phentermine-topiramate** (brand name: Qsymia) is a combination of a classic weight-loss drug (phentermine) and an anticonvulsant (topiramate), approved by the FDA in 2012. It works to lessen appetite, but due to its amphetamine-like effects, there is a risk of the drug becoming habit forming.

> » Possible side effects include increased heart rate and blood pressure, insomnia, nervousness, constipation, taste changes, tingling in hands and feet, dry mouth, and dizziness, among others. Patients are advised not to take it if pregnant or wanting to get pregnant because topiramate increases risk of birth defects.

You can also find phentermine (Adipex-P, Lomaira) by itself instead of in combination with topiramate. Approved by the FDA in 2016, this drug is generally prescribed for short-term use only. It works by suppressing appetite. The dosage is intentionally low due to risk of substance abuse. Possible side effects include irregular heartbeat, panic, dry mouth, insomnia, diarrhea, delirium, psychosis, and heart failure, among others.

To qualify for any of these FDA-approved weight-loss drugs, candidates must have a BMI of 30 or higher, or a BMI of 27 or higher and a weight-related health problem like sleep apnea, type 2 diabetes, or high blood pressure. *Ironically, many overweight people do not qualify for these prescriptions due to already high blood pressure or sleep apnea, both of which can be made worse by these medications.* The average weight loss from these drugs ranges from 3 to 9 percent of excess body weight over a period of six to twelve months. However, more information is needed to understand the long-term safety and efficacy of these medications. We do know that most weight loss occurs in the first six months after starting the medication, plateauing from there.

Unfortunately, like diets, weight-loss drugs seem to be a Band-Aid: temporarily helpful for some but ineffective in treating the deeper issues of metabolic disease. Most studies that have been done of these FDA-approved drugs are brief and underwhelming. A twenty-four-week study of orlistat from 2011, with a sample size of eighty people with BMI over 30, showed an average weight loss of 10 pounds among those who took 120 milligrams of the drug three times per day versus the 2.5-pound weight loss among those who took the placebo. Loose and oily stools were reported as a common side effect. The other prescription drugs were similarly tested and with comparable results (minus that particularly icky side effect). As you can see, studies like this may vouch for the short-term effects of the drug, but they don't report how the users fared in the long run.

There have been a few longer-term studies of weight-loss medications. One such US study of lorcaserin, published in the *New England Journal of Medicine* in 2018, followed a sample size of twelve thousand people for forty months. Tam Fry of Britain's National Obesity Forum hailed the drug as the potentially "holy grail" of weight-loss medicine because, on average, patients lost 9 pounds (4 kilograms) during those forty months without damage to their heart valves.

Healthy heart valves are great, and highly recommended. But 9 pounds for a severely obese person—is it even worth it? At my highest set point of 238, I would have been happy to get down to 229, but I still would have had a long way to go to get to a healthy BMI. And for the cost of the pill, which may or may not be out of pocket, that's not a very good deal. Let's do some math here: in that same year, a prescription for Belviq, the brand name for lorcaserin, cost approximately $250 per month. Multiply that by forty months (the average number of months that the test subjects participated to lose the average 9 pounds) . . . that's $10,000! That's $1,111.11 a pound!

Don't Cut Your Nose Off to Spite Your Face

My grandmother, who grew up in the small town of Cody, Wyoming, told me that girls in her generation swallowed live tape worms to lose weight. The science behind this repulsive practice hypothesized that tapeworms would eat your extra calories, leading to weight loss (with many unpleasant side effects ranging from digestive issues and bacterial infections to serious illness). Whether my grandmother's story is true or not, it is a disgusting and fascinating anecdote, one that I have gleefully enjoyed telling, adding in my own gruesome details over the years, and goes to show that some people will do nearly anything to be thin.

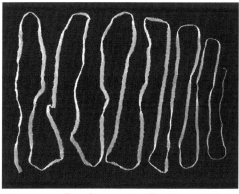
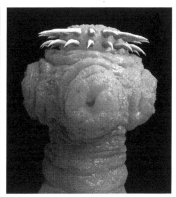

Tapeworm (length range 1 millimeter – 50 feet)   *Tapeworm head (scolex)*

Personally, I couldn't imagine swallowing a live tapeworm, or even a pill that has a tapeworm egg in it. It's just too gross. Not that I am above weight-loss experimentation. I've tried many things in my day.

Nicotine gum was an effective appetite suppressant, and chewing it was a good substitute for chewing (and swallowing) real food (even though you are actually supposed to "park" the gum and not chew too long), but it made my mouth taste like dirt, and I worried too much about addiction to stay with it for long. HCG (human chorionic gonadotropin, commonly known as human growth hormones) injections suppressed my appetite to support an extreme starvation diet; like all low-calorie diets, it was unsustainable, and undergoing daily injections in my abdomen or thigh for the rest of my days wasn't exactly viable. In the mid-1990s, I took fen-phen, when it was all the rage. It was fairly easy to get (both legally and not), and practically everyone I knew, even the skinny minis, were popping those little blue-and-white saviors.

In 1993, I was about to get married. Like so many soon-to-be brides, I wanted to look amazing in my form-fitting, delicately hand-beaded wedding dress. I dreamed of floating down the aisle on a cloud of love and thinness, while the 450 guests oohed and aahed at my angular beauty. (Yes, you read that right: 450 guests.) *Thirty pounds should do it,* I thought. I had five months to hit my goal before walking down the aisle.

The doctor who gave me the fen-phen prescription had a frustrating protocol. Each of her patients was required to lose 10 pounds *per month* in order to "earn" the next month's prescription. This was the mandate across the board, whether you were 200, 500, or a mere 167 pounds as I was. I think she was worried about getting sued, which as it turns out, was a valid fear; when fen-phen lost its FDA approval a few years later in 1997 (long after I'd ended my brief stint on the drug), several class action lawsuits were filed against the drug for causing permanent heart valve damage and pulmonary hypertension. I think my doctor thought she would appear less negligent in prescribing this amphetamine cocktail if she showed extra due diligence in her mandatory monthly weight-loss requirements. But she applied them across the board, without regard to individual needs. It worked. I was extra driven to lose the weight and stay on the drug!

"Take it first thing in the morning," the doctor told me, "or you'll never get to sleep."

She was absolutely right. Ask anyone, and they'll tell you that being on fen-phen is like being on crystal meth (not that I've ever tried meth). The euphoria was stupendous. I was not hungry at all and had an incredible amount of energy. Food just didn't seem interesting; it tasted as it did when I had a bad cold—like nothing at all! Put a piece of chocolate cake or a salad in front of me—it was all the same to me, so if I had to eat, I'd eat the salad. In fact, I was so unoccupied by appetite that I had to set a timer on my clock to remind myself to eat. Three small bites and I was full.

I lost weight. And I lost my mind.

The first week on fen-phen, I literally didn't sleep a wink. A week without sleep can do all kinds of strange things to a person, and I engaged in all kinds of bizarre and out-of-character behavior, such as methodically scrubbing the back of the toilet with a toothbrush at two in the morning. Picture a young version of the retired widow from *Requiem for a Dream*, alone in her apartment, watching self-help TV, popping pills, and grinding her teeth. That was me on fen-phen.

Thanks to my morning dose, I didn't feel tired after that first week, despite those sleepless nights. But outside of the freaky laser-focused cleaning binges, I couldn't concentrate and was super grouchy and jittery. Usually I'm an attentive driver, but a month or so after starting fen-phen, I drove straight through a red light at a busy four-way intersection during morning rush hour. I simply forgot to stop. It was a miracle that I didn't kill anyone, including myself!

On fen-phen I quickly became the worst bridezilla you can imagine. Think of the show *Bridezillas*, featuring beautiful young women with perfect skin, starving themselves and screaming at their mothers. That was me. Except that instead of being on the nuptial version of drunkorexia, a.k.a. the "white wine diet," I was on speed.

On top of the wedding prep, I was working full time, and I started making a bunch of errors, as well as lashing out at my fiancé and generally being a monster. It didn't matter—all I cared about was my wedding dress fitting, cinching in that bodice a couple extra inches. And I felt powerful. I remember speed-walking down a downtown sidewalk, passing people sitting at restaurants' outside tables and thinking, *You are eating all those French fries? Weakling. I don't even care about those anymore.* After a lifetime of believing I was fat because I was weak willed, the sensation of total self-control was a fantastic power trip.

Yet there were brief moments where I'd come to, as though waking from a dream, and I'd suddenly realize how awful I'd been acting. I'd think, *You'd better tuck it in, or you're not going to get married at all.* But then I'd quickly rationalize my behavior: *Being a little bit nuts is a hallowed bridal tradition. Everyone has stress before their wedding. I am going to look amazing.*

I would have done anything to have one memory of the wedding, of me in that dress, in which I felt dainty and light, pretty and petite, like a model in a bridal magazine. Yet under my French manicure, my nails were peeling, and my skin was ashy. I was finding my hair in clumps in the shower drain. But the weight fell off me like magic. I lost 26 of the desired 30 pounds, and yet all I could think walking down the aisle was, *If only I could have lost another 4 pounds.* I was happy to be marrying my husband, don't get me wrong. But I would have been happier as a size 4.

Remembering this now makes me sad. How focused I was on what I believed to be my imperfections, so much so that I was willing to sacrifice my sanity. I wanted to be someone else, lanky and willowy, with overly prominent collar bones. But I was just me, only a bit thinner. My mind-set and attitudes about myself and my body hadn't changed along with my weight; even if I'd met my goal weight, I'm sure I would have still been disappointed, still wished that I'd lost another 5 pounds. Looking back, I can see that I was a beautiful bride—I just didn't know it. And I now realize that my husband would've been happy to marry me whether I lost the 30 pounds or not—he put an engagement ring on the bigger version of me, after all!

Month 3, my doctor refused to refill my fen-phen prescription. I was struggling to eat even 500 calories a day but had only lost 2 pounds for the month, which did not meet her 10-pound requirement. I decided I'd show her and bought another two month's supply from a work friend who had been taking them and had a surplus. Those last two months (before tying the knot) I only lost an additional 4 pounds. Fortunately, I ran out of fen-phen just after the wedding and I made no further attempts to obtain additional pills. What with the mood swings, the insomnia, and the negative impact on my work and relationships, I realized that it was not a sustainable weight-management method. (I will admit, I missed the euphoria and feelings of being powerful and in control.) Within two months, I'd gained every pound back, plus three extra for good measure.

Whether you have tried illegal or prescription drugs, or nicotine or alcohol, to overcome obesity, chances are that, given the laundry list of nasty side effects, you have not been able to find a drug that is sustainable for long-term use. Some of us are still searching for the magic pill, but I fear we are a long way away from that elusive discovery. I do hope that the hardworking scientists and doctors, and the brave test subjects, continue their quest to better understand the complex miracle of weight loss, and that someday they will find a better medicine to treat it. Until then, I think we need to consider other options.

CHAPTER 4

Cutting through the Bullshit

Perfection is the enemy of progress.
—Winston Churchill

After I finished graduate school in Louisville, Kentucky, I moved to Phoenix, Arizona, to take a job as an administrator in a methadone clinic, which is essentially a center that dispenses medication to combat opioid dependence. Opioids include illegal drugs like heroin, as well as legal prescription-based painkillers like hydrocodone (Vicodin) and oxycodone (OxyContin). These types of drugs are highly addictive, and many users can't stop using them cold turkey. My job was to make sure everything ran smoothly at the clinic behind the scenes (administratively), supporting the clinicians in their collective mission to help drug users overcome their addiction.

Working at such a clinic had never been my dream exactly. But fresh out of school, I was idealistic and desperate for money, and besides that, this was the only job offer that quickly came my way. The clinic, located in a less-than-desirable area, was almost an hour's drive from my house. *What the hell*, I figured. *I'll stay a couple months until something better comes along.* I stayed for nearly seven years. To date, it was the toughest job I have ever had.

The methadone clinic was a clear departure from the sheltered life I'd lived up until then. Other than observing *mostly* minor recreational drug use in college, I had not been exposed to hard-core illicit drug use or drug addicts, and I'd had no reason to think too hard about whether I held any prejudices against this population. I quickly discovered that I did, in fact, subconsciously stereotype drug addicts. I was shocked to find that the methadone clients were not the indigent, uneducated, dirty, society-fringe dwellers I'd apparently assumed they would be. But I learned in my years at the clinic that addiction has no boundaries—it cuts across race, gender, religion, sexual orientation, socioeconomic status, and education.

I met all kinds of people there: the disabled veteran, the PhD candidate, the stay-at-home mom, the former professional athlete, the emergency room doctor, the high school senior, and the general contractor. These were people who were struggling, who wanted to kick the habit—otherwise, they wouldn't have been there. Most of them were genuinely working hard to get better. But many, from my naïve perspective, just weren't working hard enough.

The clinical director—I'll call him José—was an amazing man, brilliant and kind and a bit socially awkward. At the beginning of my time at the clinic, I would seek him out to talk after work hours, and we would have rich debates about life, health, family, and of course addiction. I would express my frustrations to him about the methadone patients, saying that I didn't think some of them put enough consistent effort into the recovery process. Frequently, he'd frustrate the hell out of me by saying, "You are trying to apply rational thinking to an irrational situation."

"But, but, but . . . ," I would argue, "the patients have the ability to change. They are *choosing* not to!" Like most twentysomethings, I saw everything in black and white, right or wrong, yes or no.

"Perhaps they do *not* have the ability, or the desire," he'd reply.

"No," I'd say, in a rush to make my point, "they do have the ability. And lots of them have the desire. I've talked with them, I know this to be true. They're just being lazy, and they don't want to give up the drugs."

"Perhaps they just do not have the wherewithal," he'd reply.

We never got anywhere in these circularly infuriating conversations. I was young and plucky, and to me the world was a welcoming, wide-open place, full of dreams yet to be realized. After all, *I* wasn't a drug addict, a choice I chose every single day. I could do it, so why couldn't they? It was easy! Just don't shoot up, right? *If you want to change*, I thought, *then just change.*

It wasn't until a few months into the job that I heard the phrase "self-medicating." Some of the patients, I learned, used drugs to cope with mental health issues like schizophrenia, bipolar disorder, anxiety, depression, or posttraumatic stress disorder. I was struck by how many of the patients had diagnosed serious mental illnesses that compounded their suffering and confounded their treatment, as well as histories of abuse, violence, and neglect. Their backgrounds and experiences were too varied to make any generalization, but I can say that most, if not all, were people in pain, with real genetic and environmental obstacles that made it challenging for them to get healthy.

During those seven years, my perspective changed. I watched people die. I watched people fight their addictions with determination and resignation. I watched people get healthy and go into recovery. Some held on, and some began using again a year, two years, five years down the road. It didn't take me long to recognize that addicts weren't just people bored on a Friday night with nothing better to do than try heroin. They were real people with strengths and weaknesses and complicated lives.

Take Lenny, for example. Lenny was a thirtysomething man who lived at home with his disabled father and worked part time as a day laborer or custodian. He'd been in and out of the clinic for years, desperate to kick his debilitating opioid habit. But his mental illness (schizophrenia) kept getting in his way. I remember one late afternoon I got paged to the primary clinic. I raced over to find Lenny standing in the single-occupancy bathroom off the waiting area, the door open wide. Screaming and clearly disoriented, he had his bare right foot propped up on the lip of the sink and a razor blade in his hand.

"They're after me!" he kept shouting, waving the blade around. "They're almost here!"

The clinicians and I tried to keep the other patients back. A social worker talked softly to Lenny, reassuring him that no one was after him, that he was having a hallucination. He ended up cutting off three of his toes before we could tackle him to the ground, his blade clattering to the ground as blood poured out onto the Saltillo tile floor.

As you can imagine, this incident scared the hell out of me. It also broke my heart: Lenny had really tried to get better. I'd seen his efforts, talked to him many times about how much work he was putting into his program, how hard he was fighting to get well. He came to the clinic regularly, participated in both individual and group sessions, and tried to stay on his antipsychotic medications in spite of their negative side effects. The desire was there; the ability was not.

I watched many people like Lenny slip through the social safety net's gaping holes. Some, though, had every opportunity and resource offered up to them on a silver platter, and they still struggled. I remember this one guy I will call Cooper, a prominent politician with a spotless record and stellar reputation. He was very intelligent and charismatic, and somehow he'd managed to hide his addiction from everyone, including his family. Many politicians and leaders like to take risks—that's how and why they get to the top. I believe that, for him, drug use was about the thrill, about fun and danger, as well as escapism. Who knows what demons were chasing him? Cooper was what we called a "high-functioning" heroin addict, and for the first few years I think he viewed treatment as another risky form of entertainment, like a game he could win if only he decided he wanted to. He just didn't seem to care all that much, or take his addiction seriously. He was doing fine, after all, with a good job and a solid place in his community. At a certain point, however, his political aspirations grew, and he decided it was time to finally get serious. After true desire came into play, he was able to recover.

Both Lenny and Cooper had the same problem: opiate drug addiction. But each struggled with it in their own unique way, and for a variety of reasons, only Cooper was able to recover. It wasn't for lack of desire or effort on Lenny's part that he couldn't; there were just so many environmental and genetic factors working against him. If anyone "deserved" to get better, it was him. Unfortunately, that's not how addiction works.

I stayed at the methadone clinic for so many years because my hope grew, rather than faded, as my black-and-white perspective on addiction softened into gray. The patients were not bad people, or lazy. Their crippling drug addiction was not all their fault. It was not black and white, right or wrong, yes or no. Getting better was not a simple one-time choice.

Cut It the Hell Out

The US National Institute on Drug Abuse has advocated a brain disease model of addiction (BDMA) since 1997. Instead of assuming that the alcoholic passed out on the city bench could get better if only he wanted to, the BDMA suggests that we should offer our compassion, look for a medical reason for his problem, and work to find a medical solution. Though the BDMA model continues to be controversial, and some experts argue it is too reductionist, it goes a long way toward getting rid of the stigma that has stood in the way of addicts' access to treatment. Yes, addicts make choices—it would be patronizing to claim otherwise. But the genetic inheritances and lifetime of experiences that converge to push an addict to order one more G&T are complex. How can we judge addicts' ability, desire, and wherewithal without knowing their full stories?

We're getting into "free will" territory here. I am not a philosopher (well, only sometimes, after a quiet morning taking in a sunrise), but it's hard to avoid being philosophical when we start discussing impulses and temptation and our ability to resist them. We Americans can't escape our Puritan roots stemming from the sixteenth and seventeenth centuries, the precept we've inherited that says our inability to resist our human needs and wants is a soul-level moral failing. At the end of the day, the body is an imperfect vessel that exists in the real world rather than on some spiritual plane, and there's only so much you can do to control and steer it. You can resist some of your impulses some of the time, and some of your impulses all of the time, but you cannot resist all the impulses all of the time.

It's easy for me to resist the impulse to freebase heroin. It is not easy for me to resist a sale at Nordstrom, a slice of carrot cake with cream cheese frosting, or a long walk with my dogs on a windy autumn day. That's just me. Everyone has impulses, and the level of choice each of us has in giving in to each impulse is up for debate. Some of your impulses might be easy for me to resist, and some of my impulses might prove no problem for you.

Still, we now know enough not to tell someone who drinks a fifth of Jack Daniel's every day for ten years to just cut it the hell out. If only it were that easy. We've come to accept that most severe alcoholics require medical intervention so that their bodies can heal enough (rather than going into cold-turkey withdrawal) for them to stand a chance at long-term recovery. This does not mean they do not have to manage their impulses and change bad habits and self-destructive behaviors—obviously they do. But they also need real, effective treatment, a means to "reset," to get them to a physical state in which recovery is possible.

So, where am I going with all this? Just as heroin or alcohol addiction is a disease, the inability to gain control over your appetite and metabolism is also a disease. Sometimes, after years of struggle with this disease, diseases that are more widely recognized and accepted, such as type 2 diabetes or high blood pressure, can manifest. I have a friend with diagnosed diabetes who refuses to take any kind of medication or receive insulin shots and instead says things like, "I know I have a problem; I just need to lose weight." Her words echo those I heard from patients in the methadone clinic year after year: "I don't want to take methadone; I will just quit heroin." She has made many real attempts to lose weight. And thus far, she has failed. She has the desire, without a doubt, and she has the wherewithal to change her behaviors for months, even years, at a time. Sometimes she loses 5 or 10 pounds. Once she even lost 50. But because she has a metabolic disease, no matter how hard she works, the weight always comes back, and the diabetes persists, leaving her feeling ill much of the time.

As one of the unlucky people who have the desire and the wherewithal but not the ability, I can tell you just how frustrating it is to be truly working hard to live a healthy lifestyle and yet still not lose weight. The thin woman running on the treadmill next to me at the gym will get credit for her efforts; I will not. I know all too well what it's like to live with the stigma that comes with being fat, an assumption that I am lazy or ignorant. Add to that the fact that employment laws don't yet fully protect obese people from discrimination. I often travel for work, and let me tell you: the heat of the passengers' glares that used to come my way as I walked down the too-narrow aisle of the airplane could microwave a 240-calorie Lean Cuisine meatloaf with mashed potatoes dinner. *God, I hope she doesn't sit next to me,* I could practically hear them thinking, as though my fatness was a personal affront.

Air travel is uncomfortable for everyone—the lack of leg room, the recycled air, the oversalted snacks, and the shared armrests. For overweight people, the discomfort is tenfold. Scratch that: a hundredfold. Those times I had the misfortune of not getting an aisle seat, and the other passengers in my row couldn't be bothered to move, I would have to squeeze past my seatmates before taking my seat, which felt, at times, like an impossible feat. My first attempt to buckle my seat belt would be fraught with worry: would I be able to get it around my belly, or would I have to endure the humiliation of asking for a seat-belt extender (or risk noncompliance with safety procedure by not wearing it). My upper thighs would spill over the edges of my seat, encroaching on my neighbor. When the beverage cart came around, I worried that people would judge me if I bought a meal or drank anything other than plain water.

Flying can be dangerous for fat people too. Before every flight, I'd put on medical-grade compression clothing. Not just socks—I'm talking about a full-on bodysuit. Let me tell you, getting into that thing was a feat on par with a Cirque du Soleil performance, at the end of which I'd feel as if I'd just run a marathon. I'd also take blood thinners, which unfortunately have a number of potential uncomfortable side effects, such as nosebleeds, dizziness, and muscle weakness, along with the more serious risk of bleeding out from minor injury. (To this day, I still toss back a couple aspirin before every flight—old habits die hard.) I underwent all of this to avoid getting a blood clot, which is a serious health concern, particularly for the obese. Deep vein thrombosis (DVT) usually occurs in the legs and can, in fact, kill you, if one of those blood clots heads north and blocks blood to the brain or lungs.

Sometimes, during one of those eleven-hour flights to South Korea or England, I'd wonder if the pain of wearing what was essentially a head-to-toe straightjacket was worth its benefit. Wherever the nylon met flesh felt like being cut with a knife. On top of that, I still felt compelled to get up every hour to stop my blood from settling in my calves, another surefire way to piss off my seatmates. And God help me if I had to use the restroom.

I was so deeply ashamed by this secret-in-plain-sight that I never talked about it with anyone, not even my husband. And I didn't want to risk my job; in my experience, career advancement in business today is correlated with the size and scope of your oversight, meaning these days you often have to go global if you want to achieve a certain level of expertise in your profession. I worried that if I said anything that had a whiff of complaint in it, or if anyone knew that air travel was excruciating both physically and emotionally for me, I could jeopardize my career. I'd be left with a few days' worth of swollen ankles—for me, the phrase "muffin top" applies not to the fat hanging over my waist but to the liquid "jelly" roll just above my shoe—only to have to do it all again to get home. I loved my career, but sometimes, after disembarking the plane, I thought about quitting just so I could avoid this pain.

All these years I have felt completely alone in my stressful travel experiences. But now I realize I wasn't. In the opening scene of her young adult novel *Fat Girl on a Plane*, Kelly Devos describes air travel anxiety for overweight people in excruciating detail: "No. You can't just buy two seats in advance. . . . One person equals one seat reservation. You can thank global terrorism for that one." Kelly Devos uses tragic humor to describe the awkward moments at the gate where the flight attendants use "judgment calls" (i.e., whether you appear too fat) to decide if a last-minute additional seat must be purchased. The anonymous writer "Your Fat Friend" discusses this phenomenon too in a post on *Medium*, entitled "What It's Like to Be That Fat Person Sitting Next to You on the Plane." She talks about the state of panic she'll be in for weeks before she has to fly somewhere for a business trip or a friend's wedding. She'll obsessively research airline policies for "passengers of size," debate whether she should wear one or two layers of Spanx, check her bag, and bring a seat-belt extender in her carry-on so no one will have another reason to complain about her. Those days leading up to her flight are always filled with dread.

What I'm trying to say is, if fat people could easily change their size, most would in a heartbeat. Anyone in his right mind would do anything to avoid that anxiety and pain, those glares and grumbles (and worse) from strangers. After years of shame, I've come to realize that obesity is not a moral deficiency, or a calorie-in, calorie-out equation. It is a symptom of an underlying physical problem in which a series of complex chemical reactions in the body drives us to maintain an above-normal set point weight through lethargy and appetite. Some see overweight people overeating—or, really, just eating—or being sedentary and think, *Just stop it* or *That person is lazy* or *They could change if they really wanted to.* As if a fat person could just flip a switch and the next day all those pounds would melt away! If only. If you have been significantly overweight for ten years or more, you know how ridiculous that notion is.

Embracing the Gut

Obviously, everyone *doesn't* know how ridiculous that is. A year ago, a friend told me about a conversation she'd overheard in the changing room of her yoga studio. This friend—I'll call her Simone—worked in the tech world as a consultant, and as such, she could control her own schedule. Her favorite yoga class was on Fridays at noon, for which she would step away from her keyboard, throw on her leggings and a ratty old T-shirt with the sleeves cut off, and head over to the studio. This studio was located in a nearby suburb made up of middle-class, upper-class, and rich households, who owned the sprawling mansions on the water with boats parked dockside down below.

This conversation took place in the changing room after a particularly sweaty class. Simone was minding her own business when one of two women—let's call her Robin—said, "I don't know why people always talk about how hard it is to lose the baby weight after a pregnancy. I mean, I did it."

The other woman didn't say anything. Out of the corner of her eye, Simone saw her shrug.

"Not saying it didn't take work," Robin continued. She was changing her clothes unhurriedly, peeling off her designer spandex to reveal a flat, Caribbean-vacation-tanned belly. "I ate right, cut gluten out of my diet entirely. I exercised, I did acupuncture. I went to the spa so I could do cycles of sauna and cold-water plunges. That really helps kick up the metabolism! I lost the weight in a couple months, no problem."

Simone had to grit her teeth to stop herself from chiming in. She knew this woman outside the studio. Robin lived in one of those sprawling mansions down by the lake, she didn't have to earn an income to support her household, and she had a full-time nanny helping raise her kids. She practiced yoga religiously, sometimes going to two classes a day, and her Instagram was full of photos of her doing pretzel-ey poses on her dock, next to her boat. On top of that, she was probably 5 feet 1 in heels and had gone into each of her pregnancies without an extra ounce of fat.

Simone, on the other hand, had gained 40 pounds while pregnant with her son a decade earlier. She'd lost 25 of those pounds, but no matter what she did, those additional 15 pounds had become her new norm. She didn't worry about her weight gain all that much; she had other concerns, such as potty training and making sure her child didn't run into oncoming traffic while also maintaining a loving marriage and working a full-time job.

In Robin's judgments I heard the echo of the words I'd spoken when I'd started at the methadone clinic. Clearly Robin blamed the mothers for not losing the baby weight. She assumed they were lazy, that they lacked desire, wherewithal, and gumption. She had managed to lose the baby weight and keep it off, after all, a choice she made every day. But she failed to recognize her own unique privilege—not just her genetic predisposition but also the support and time her life afforded her, which she could devote to fitness and maintaining her figure. This convergence of factors had allowed her to lose that baby weight, no problem. Not everyone is so lucky. And also, maybe we shouldn't devote all of our time to our appearance; maybe it is not healthy to obsess so completely, as Robin did, over our fitness and looks. Kelley Gunter, in her book *You Have Such a Pretty Face*, says it best: "Negotiating life about who we are based on how we look is like being Homecoming Queen of crazy town."

It is difficult to separate obesity's health concerns from its societal stigma. I wonder what my life would have been like if I had become overweight when "fat shaming" was a common phrase, if how to reject it had been a part of the cultural conversation. Would I have spent so much time worrying, starving, and feeling ashamed? Would I have accepted myself as I was? There's no way to know. But I do know that, when I started regular air travel, there were no internet posts by bloggers like Your Fat Friend, where I might have found fellow overweight travelers going through similar airplane experiences. If there had been, I might not have felt so alone.

Oh, how much time I have wasted on sweating (literally and figuratively) over being fat. Before my surgery, I figure that, on a good day, I spent 40 percent of my brain's processing capacity on something related to my weight. Let's say 10 percent of the sweating went toward what people thought about my fat (BRUTAL). The next 10 percent of my mind space was spent sweating over how negatively I felt within my body hour to hour (SOUL CRUSHING and DEMORALIZING). And as I aged, the remaining 20 percent (which, honestly, increased a few percentage points each year) was spent sweating over my health (or lack thereof). I literally felt I could be diagnosed with something awful—cancer, heart disease—at any moment and that I would have no one to blame but myself. I wish I were one of those people who could say, "I have no regrets." But I am not. I want that mind space back. I should've been using that space to live, dream, innovate, love, and come up with unselfish acts to carry out, but I wasted it on an obsessive and unavoidable GIANT—my weight. Forty percent compounded over thirty years! I shudder to think of it.

These days, body positivity is a cultural phenomenon. There are even overweight people on TV and in the movies! Gone (I hope) are the days of *Shallow Hall*, *Bridget Jones's Diary* (Renee Zellweger is supposed to be overweight? Get real!), or *Love Actually*, a movie that supposes we're all wonderfully surprised when the prime minister, played by the floppy-haired Hugh Grant, finds his sweet catering manager to be a babe even though her ribcage doesn't appear in sharp relief through her shirt. I would be lying if I didn't admit that I loved a couple of these movies and watched them over and again, but they perpetuate stereotypes that are in desperate need of breaking.

In current rom-coms, cultural commentary, and satire, fat-related story lines often focus less on dropping pounds and more on overcoming shame as a path to happiness. Amy Schumer's 2018 comedy *I Feel Pretty* is one example of this. Of course, the protagonist has to sustain a traumatic brain injury to feel pretty, but the movie's point is that self-esteem is a state of mind, not a dress size. While the movie has been criticized for being fat shaming, and Schumer, the "fat girl," clearly has a normal body mass index (BMI), I do believe the movie is genuinely meant to be uplifting and funny, providing us with a new message about weight and self-esteem. Other shows and movies serve to hold a magnifying glass to fat shaming, such as AMC's *Dietland*, which explores a wide range of current female issues, including unrealistic body standards. Another example is Netflix's *Dumplin'*, in which an overweight teenager signs up for a beauty pageant against her mother's wishes. Granted, we still call these actresses with normal BMIs "brave" simply for acting and living in their own bodies, but it's a step in the right direction!

Then there's the good work of body-positive writers, bloggers, and activists, including Lindy West, Roxane Gay, "fat, brown, queer" Caleb Luna, Ashleigh Shackelford, Leah Vernon, and Bethany Rutter; plus-size fashionistas Jessica Hinkle, Cat Polivoda, Kelvin Davis, and Alysse Dalessandro; and "Bad Fat Broads" podcasters Ariel Woodson and KC Slack. Blogger Virgie Tovar started the hashtag #LoseHateNotWeight in an effort to destigmatize being overweight. And though books on losing weight still dominate the market for books about being fat, there are a growing number of titles out there such as *Two Whole Cakes: How to Stop Dieting and Learn to Love Your Body* (by Lesley Kinzel), *The Body Is Not an Apology: The Power of Radical Self-Love* (by Sonya Renee Taylor), and *Fat Activism: A Radical Social Movement* (by Charlotte Cooper).

Click through the hundreds of TEDx videos on YouTube, and you'll find talks like "Why It's OK to Be Fat" by Golda Poretsky and "I Am Fat—How to Be Confident and Love Your Body Size" by Victoria Welsby, which ends with fat-and-proud Welsby dancing on stage in a shiny blue bikini. Mainstream magazines are even getting on board—*Cosmopolitan* featured a plus-size model on its cover (Tess Holliday stunned on the October 2018 issue)—and major retailers like Everlane and Topshop have started to include normal-looking models in their catalogs. Even legacy brands have gotten in on the fat-acceptance trend. Take Dove, for example, whose "Real Beauty" campaign has women of all shapes and sizing in lingerie. Showing models who might look like the product's actual customers? What a novel idea!

This fat-embracing movement is wonderful, and a long time coming. We're in a moment of sweeping cultural change, and I am the first to wish fat shaming good riddance. That fact puts me in a somewhat awkward position, though, given that I am writing a book advocating a medical procedure for weight loss. The very last thing I want to do is reinforce the stigma that has plagued me for my entire adult life. So I've struggled with how to think and talk about two seemingly opposing ideas: (1) Thinness is not morally superior to fatness. (2) Sometimes, for some people, it's a good idea to lose weight.

You can be fat and healthy. There are some fat people in the world whose adipose tissue doesn't cause them any trouble. And if they can manage the stress of belonging to a marginalized group, if they can love themselves in the face of discrimination and prejudice, and if they can move freely and feel good in their bodies, then more power to them. They do not need to consider bariatric surgery.

Unfortunately, for many of us, fatness comes with health problems like type 2 diabetes and high blood pressure. These conditions have serious long-term implications. Type 2 diabetes, for example, develops if the body produces too little insulin or resists insulin, and it can lead to kidney disease, nerve damage, heart disease, hearing problems, and more. The Centers for Disease Control and Prevention (CDC) estimates that thirty million Americans currently have diabetes (about one in ten people) and 90 to 95 percent of them have type 2 diabetes. Heart disease occurs when arteries become filled with plaque, restricting blood flow, which can cause heart attack, stroke, or congestive heart failure. Heart disease is the leading cause of death in the country today. In fact, according to Harvard University Health, it takes the life of one in three Americans. And that's for both genders: the average age for a first heart attack is sixty-five for men and seventy-two for women.

Being overweight can also lead to real physical discomfort. I'm talking about the horror of plane rides, yes, but also about the more mundane difficulties involved in our everyday life: exercising, getting in and out of the car, and even tying shoes. More than one person has told me their come-to-Jesus moment happened the instant they realized they could no longer get down on the floor to play with their child. Then there are swollen ankles and overwhelming hunger and shortness of breath and lethargy. For many of us who are overweight, there is real day-to-day discomfort and pain.

Obese people shouldn't have to find themselves in a state of emergency before they can get help. We shouldn't have to be near death for the medical profession to take us seriously. We shouldn't have to waste our precious lives on diet, exercise, and drugs that don't work, only to die too young of heart disease or diabetes.

Society punishes people who have diseases that society does not like. What is the root of this thinking? We have to question why some diseases are acceptable and others are not. No one would give someone a hard time for using an inhaler for asthma or getting a torn ACL fixed. Do we punish those with type 2 diabetes because we're afraid of it? Is it simply a human tendency to push away or demonize that which we do not fully understand? Or do we think the people who have conditions like heart disease are to blame and thus deserve what they get? We have much more compassion for drug and alcohol addiction than we used to. Hopefully we are moving toward increased understanding and empathy for those with unhealthy extra weight and weight-related conditions.

In order to do that, we have to accept that the issue of obesity goes far beyond personal habits and choices, that weight is not just an issue of ability, desire, and wherewithal. We must believe in obese people's right to legitimate medical intervention. **Bariatric surgery should be a real option for those of us whose lives are limited because of our weight, who are experiencing ill health, or have been warned by trustworthy doctors that we are heading in that direction.**

CHAPTER 5

Cut to the Bone

Tomorrow is the most important thing in life.
Comes into us at midnight very clean. It's perfect
when it arrives and it puts itself in our hands. It
hopes we've learned something from yesterday.
—John Wayne

What do you do when you realize that everything you have done, everything you have been faithful to for years, hasn't worked? What happens when you decide that you're finally done blaming yourself?

I remember being a kid and hearing my elders talk about where they were when they heard that John F. Kennedy had been assassinated. It seemed strange to me at the time that somehow everyone could recall that exact moment. But for us younger folks, most of us remember what we were doing when we got the news of the airplanes crashing into the Twin Towers on September 11, 2001. I was standing in a Seattle conference room when someone rushed in and turned on the TV, which was showing replay after replay of this catastrophe on every channel. I was listening to the radio on

Highway 101 in Phoenix when I heard that Princess Diana had been killed in 1997, and I remember the feeling of my shoes hitting the sidewalk in Tokyo in 2016 when someone yelled on the street, "The Artist, Prince, is dead."

These are the kinds of memories that stick. In the same way, I remember the sun shining on the leaves of a birch tree through my windshield and the smell of my warm leather seats the morning I sat frozen in my car in the parking lot outside my doctor's office. I'd just left a routine dermatology appointment. A nurse and I had been going through the usual check-in, and she'd asked about any health changes since my last appointment. She paused for a moment and then, off topic and unsolicited, casually said, "The chances of losing weight at our age are very low." She then proceeded to rattle off statistics about weight loss and health in our fifties, as if she'd just returned from a continuing education unit course on the subject. She clearly knew what she was talking about, and although she seemed well intentioned, all I wanted to do, as she spoke, was RUN AWAY!

As statistics continued to pour out of her, I started to feel stone-in-the-pit-of-my-stomach, about-to-vomit-and-cry sick. Afterward, I could barely make it through the rest of my appointment. *Keep it together, Jamie,* I kept thinking, trying to take deep breaths. Why was I having this visceral reaction? I already knew most of what she was saying anyway—she wasn't offering up any real surprises. Anyway, I'd heard it all before from doctors and had become numb, if not defensive, to the "you need to lose some weight" comments. Was I caught off guard because I had not expected this impromptu conversation from the dermatologist's nurse?

Whatever the reason, it was in that instant that I finally realized I was likely never going to lose the 80-pound fat suit I had been wearing for the past fifteen years. Up until that moment, I'd always had hope. Moreover, I had always known deep inside that I would be thin again someday. My sister, the love of my life and my biggest champion, knew it too. She had rooted for me with unwavering faith, believing with her whole heart that I would inevitably triumph.

I am not a crier. My children have told me they think it's odd that they have rarely seen me shed a tear. It's not good or bad; it is just the way I am. But let me tell you: on this particular day, I made up for lost time. After my appointment, sitting there in my car, with the sun shining down on the birch tree, I sobbed inconsolably. What would living the rest of my life at 238 pounds mean for my longevity, my health, and my family and friends?

I learned a long time ago in my work that activity does not equal accomplishment. I try to live by this motto. Yet here I was, staring at fifteen years of unproductive weight loss. All those early mornings I sacrificed drinking coffee in bed with my husband for a torturous three-mile run. The nights I watched my kids enjoy my husband's delicious mac and cheese while I picked at a romaine salad. The social events I'd opted out of for fear of breaking my diet, the hours at the gym, the daily pangs of hunger. What if I had stopped this wild goose chase years ago? What if I had spent all that time being overweight and happy? Where had I gone wrong? How the hell did I get here?

For the first time, I let myself sit with the full magnitude of the sorrow, the fear, and the regret. Over an hour later, I was still sitting there in my car, watching the birch leaves sway as the light shifted. I could no longer play the "what if" game: What if I just hadn't eaten that one bite of chocolate that one time while slogging through that three-month diet? What if I'd run five miles instead of three? What if I'd been even more religious about Weight Watchers, Atkins, and Optifast? In those moments, I could finally clearly see that for me, diet and exercise alone was simply not going to work.

Finally, I turned the key in the ignition and drove home. For the next few days, my normal jovial mood was replaced with muted anger. I knew that my next step would be getting my head around the fact that I was going to be heavy for whatever life I had left. I decided that I would never diet again. I would do my best to live a healthy life to the extent that my body allowed, and that was that. I'd let go of my dreams of renewing my wedding vows on a Hawaiian beach in a size 8 dress. My thirty-year struggle was over. I should have felt relieved on some level, but I didn't. I was stoic. Controlled on the outside but batshit crazy angry within.

Cutting Your Emotions

Many of you may be familiar with the Kübler-Ross model of the five stages of grief, which first appeared in Dr. Elisabeth Kübler-Ross's 1969 book *On Death and Dying.* These five stages are denial, anger, bargaining, depression, and acceptance, but not necessarily in that order. This model has been used and altered to describe many common phenomena in the human experience, including change.

As the vice president of a human resources department, when there's a company-wide reorganization or the introduction of a new methodology or system, I'm brought in to help people prepare themselves for the emotional and behavioral components that can accompany upheaval. This work is called organizational change management, and I teach this eight-step model of change:

STAGES OF CHANGE

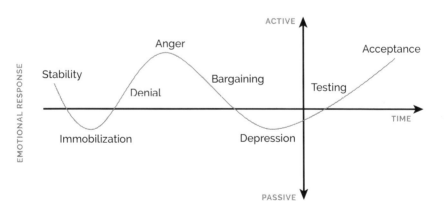

- **Stability:** Status quo—life as usual.
- **Immobilization:** When you learn about the impending change, you are in shock and unable to respond.

- **Denial:** As the impact of the change sinks in, you refuse to accept that it's really going to happen.
- **Anger:** When it becomes clear that the change is likely, you have strong feelings of anger and resistance.
- **Bargaining:** You experience a spike of energy, and you try to bargain your way back to at least some aspects of the previous state.
- **Depression:** When it becomes clear there is no going back, you go through a period of depression and despondency.
- **Testing:** You start testing ways to cope with and adjust to the change.
- **Acceptance:** You come to accept the change and move on to your "new normal."

Why is this change model important? It helps us understand the impact of and emotions involved with change, giving us a way to recognize and name our own behaviors and the behavior of others. Hopefully, being aware of this change model allows us to see where we might get stuck, giving us the ability to cut ourselves and others some slack, and seek help if we need it.

When I teach this model, I like to emphasize two main points:

- Change is not linear. Not everyone starts at the stability stage, working through each stage in order until they reach acceptance. Some people experience only some of these stages, and there is no clear time limit, schedule, or order (beyond the arbitrary one you might impose on yourself or others). Acceptance too may come and go; it's common to get to acceptance, revert, and then reach it again.
- There is no right way or wrong way to deal with change (though some approaches can be more productive than others). Each of us moves through change differently.

Can you think of a difficult change you have experienced? Using this model as a basic guide, ask yourself,

- What emotions did you experience? When? Why?
- What behaviors did you exhibit based on your feelings?
- Did you eventually accept the change and reach a new status quo in the timeframe that you wanted? Why or why not?
- What did you do well? What could you have done differently?

Thinking about the answers to these questions can give you insight into your emotional response to change—how you might have shown strength in certain instances and gotten stuck in others. In the long run, pondering these questions may help you better adapt to future changes (bariatric surgery being one of those).

After that conversation with the nurse, I stayed in the anger stage for a long, long time. I was furious that I had "wasted" years of my life dieting and exercising to no avail, and I was angry that a healthy body mass index (BMI) wasn't in the cards for me. Eventually I moved into the immobilization stage, feeling plain numb. Everything I thought I knew, everything I thought I could count on happening "someday," just wasn't coming, and I needed some time to grieve that fact. Then I went back to anger, then depression, then immobilization, then round and round again. After a while, I shifted into a mournful form of acceptance, and I announced to my sister that the fight was over. It was what it was. I was done talking, I was done fighting, I was just done.

If you are very, very lucky, a new door will open at just such a time. I was lucky.

My mom, whom my sister and I affectionately call the "News Hawk" or just the "Hawk" because she knows everything that is happening around the world (sometimes even before it happens), called to tell me about a news segment on a new weight-loss procedure she'd seen. I was a bit surprised, as this wasn't something she would usually highlight or endorse, nor had we ever discussed *any* type of surgery for weight loss. I barely listened as she talked about "quilting the stomach," and she seemed confused by my complete lack of enthusiasm. A couple days later, I looked up the procedure, but I couldn't find credible medical professionals who endorsed it, so I chalked our conversation and my internet search up to more time wasted on the illusion of meaningful weight loss. I scolded myself for even being curious.

Still, my mother's phone call stayed with me, and I realized I had taught the people close to me to share new weight-loss ideas with me whenever they stumbled upon them. Their intentions were good, had always been good, but I was over it. It was time to set everyone straight. Calling my sister seemed to be a good place to start. "Listen, Jo," I said, "I know you love me and want me to be healthy and happy. But I need you to stop searching for ways to help me lose weight." I was back to being angry, filled with years of pent-up diet-failure frustration, which I proceeded to take out on the person to whom I was closest. I wanted everyone to just shut up! Most of all, I wanted to be left where I was: without hope. I was exhausted, tired of pinning my future on the next fix only to be disappointed.

My sister surprised me by staying calm in the face of my barrage. Once I'd exhausted myself, she said, "Have you looked into 'real' bariatric surgery?"

I paused, taken aback. After a moment, I said, "What are you talking about? Bariatric surgery is for the super obese. It's a cop-out and it's dangerous and HELL, NO, I haven't looked into it!" I hung up but kept the conversation going in my head. *At 39 BMI, I probably wouldn't even qualify,* I thought. *And letting someone cut into my abdomen and remove a part of my stomach or rearrange my guts as a solution? No, thank you. My problem is not nearly that dire, and I am certainly not going to that extreme.*

I didn't know it at the time, but I had finally found the answer I had been searching for most of my adult life—thanks, of course, to my beloved sister.

Cut Your Losses

Change is really hard. But what about the cost—financial, physical, and spiritual—of *not* changing?

My brother-in-law loves his spreadsheets. By day, he uses them for project management in the semiconductor industry. By night, he budgets and analyzes every household dollar spent on his spreadsheets— thereby driving my sister crazy. But while I've listened to her vent about his data-driven behavior, I know she secretly gives him credit for his thorough and reasoned nature. He is an analytic type of guy who harnesses the power of business intelligence (BI) data to run a well-managed life.

If I had tracked my spending as did my brother-in-law during the years that I was overweight, I'm pretty sure I would have been astounded to see how much was going to things like specialized diet foods, unused gym memberships, extra medical costs, and plus-size clothing. Obesity can be expensive. And the older we get, the greater the medical price tag.

Americans give billions of dollars to the diet industry machine every year. And every year, the typical dieter makes four attempts to lose weight. Let's say the average cost of a gym membership is $55 per month, or $660 a year, and the average cost of a specialty meal plan is $12 per day, or $4,380 per year. Then there's the other day-to-day costs of obesity, including

- plus-size clothing (much more expensive than "regular" sizes);
- X-wide shoes (more expensive than normal);
- large, gas-guzzling cars (a more comfortable fit);
- household services that you find difficult to do on your own because of your weight (yard maintenance, house-cleaning, or other personal household help for you, your children, or even your pets);

- copays to doctors for visits related to weight;
- copays on labs related to weight;
- pharmacy copays on medication related to weight;
- other health- and weight-loss-related services, such as therapy, acupuncture, hypnosis, yoga classes, and personal training (all of which may or may not lead to life-changing results in the end);
- compression socks to improve blood flow and prevent swelling;
- seat-belt extensions; and
- additional or upgraded airline seats.

It is undeniable that obese people have to spend more money on basic life maintenance than those with a normal BMI. How much additional money will you *really* spend this year because you are overweight?

Then there's the cost to your health. According to the Centers for Disease Control and Prevention, the health consequences of obesity are

- high blood pressure,
- high cholesterol,
- type 2 diabetes,
- heart disease,
- stroke,
- gallbladder disease,
- osteoarthritis,
- breathing problems, including sleep apnea,
- some types of cancer,
- emotional pain and stress, and
- physical pain and difficulty moving.

From data gathered from 2006 to 2013, it is estimated that non-obese people's expenditures on medical care increases approximately $197 per year, while obese individuals' spending grows each year by a whopping $3,429! And on a national scale, the spending is going up as well. Out of the $342.2 billion of total medical costs, a growing percentage is devoted to treating obesity-related illnesses, from 20.6 percent in 2005 to 25.5 percent in 2010 to 28.2 percent in 2013.

Another name for the cost of not changing is pain, or dissatisfaction. Are you spending your hard-earned cash on obesity-related items like seat-belt extensions, compression socks, and doctor bills? Are you worried about or experiencing type 2 diabetes, sleep apnea, high blood pressure, or cancer? Then you might be ready for a change.

What does it take to really change? Over the years, I've presented the Formula for Change, first attributed to David Gleicher by Richard Beckhard in the 1970s (modified later by Dannemiller), to leadership teams and employees going through major shifts. It goes like this: **C = (ABD) > X, where C = change, A = the status quo dissatisfaction, B = a desired clear state, D = practical steps to the desired state, and X = the cost of the change.**

Another way to say it is this: **CHANGE** occurs when the **DISSATISFACTION** of staying the same multiplied by the **VISION** of a desired new state multiplied by clear **FIRST** steps for moving forward is greater than or outweighs the **RESISTANCE** to stay the same (pain and cost that makes us resist change may be financial or may also involve other tangibles/intangibles).

$$C = D \times V \times F > R$$

Change happens when *the products of . . .*
- **Dissatisfaction** with the current state
- **Vision** of a more compelling possible future, and practical
- **First steps** toward a different future

are *greater than* the
- **Resistance**, the pain, or cost of change

For those of you who need a basic multiplication refresher, remember that multiplying anything by 0 equals zilch, zippo, nada—zero. So if you have extreme dissatisfaction with the status quo/current state (**D for DISSATISFACTION**) and a compelling vision of the future (**V for VISION**), but no clear first steps for moving forward (**F for FIRST STEPS**), you will not change. Or if you have extreme **DISSATISFACTION** but have no **VISION** for an alternative situation, you will not change. And of course no **DISSATISFACTION** equals no motivation—so that's a nonstarter. If any of the first three parts of the equation is missing, the whole thing equals 0.

So what if you can assign some value for **D**, **V**, and **F**? That's great, but if it isn't greater than/doesn't outweigh the cost of change or your **RESISTANCE** to the change, change will not occur.

At that moment outside the dermatologist's office, I had plenty of dissatisfaction and a vision for the future, but all of a sudden, the steps for moving forward were a big fat zero (pun intended). Dieting didn't work. Exercise didn't work. Drugs didn't work. Sitting there in the car, I just couldn't see a way forward. Realizing that *my* change equation equaled zero and that I was going nowhere sent me on a rollercoaster ride of anger, immobilization, depression, and acceptance.

Then my sister gave me a possible new first step for a healthier life: seeking out bariatric surgery. All of a sudden, I had the dissatisfaction, the vision, and a potential path forward, all of which very clearly outweighed the cost of staying the same. My change equation looked something like this:

Change	=	Dissatisfaction	✖	Vision	✖	First Steps	>	Resistance
Substantial and Sustainable Weight Loss		30 years of emotional, mental, and physical pain of being overweight		A healthier, longer life. Skinny ankles. Easier travel. Even better sex!		Setting up three interviews with bariatric surgeons to explore options and outcomes		Fear of surgery. Cost of surgery. Time off work.

After finally coming to an epiphany about my weight, I spent the next year doing in-depth research and interviewing doctors and patients throughout the United States and abroad. I walked around ruminating on all the time and money I'd wasted, all the harsh judgment I'd endured—both my own and other people's. I continued a new bumpy ride of anger to acceptance and back again on my new path toward bariatric surgery, making pit stops at all the other stages along the way. The anger—the D in the Formula for Change—grew and grew, and what started as a simmer became a boil. I wanted to yell at anyone who would listen: I would *not* die young. I would *not* allow everyone who loves me to watch me die slowly because of health complications related to my obesity. *Stop lying!* I wanted to tell the diet industry, and *Shut up and open your eyes!* I wanted to say to all of those doctors and other health professionals who'd keep telling me over and over again that all I had to do was diet and exercise. *Mind your own damn self!* I wanted to say to anyone who looked at me sideways. I'd had more than enough.

It is time, I told myself, *to cut my gut.*

Where are *you* in this equation? My guess is that, if you're reading this book, you or someone you love has suffered a meaningful amount of pain surrounding their weight. Maybe, like me, you've had a vision of a healthier future, and you've tried and failed, then rewritten the steps for getting there, over and over again. How can *you* alter the equation to make real change occur? Perhaps it's time to consider bariatric surgery.

PART
TWO

CHAPTER 6

Cut to the Chase

Remember, tomorrow is promised to no one.
—Walter Payton

Obesity doesn't have a one-size-fits-all cause, so it doesn't have a one-size-fits-all solution. Bariatric surgery is definitely not right for everyone. Like most surgeries, there are health risks associated with going under the knife, including death. But according to the Centers for Disease Control and Prevention, the death rate due to complications from general surgical care is on the decline, and the American Society for Metabolic and Bariatric Surgery (ASMBS) Bariatric Centers of Excellence database shows that the risk of death within the first thirty days following bariatric surgery averages 0.13 percent, or approximately one out of one thousand patients. This rate is considerably less than most other operations, including gallbladder and hip replacement surgery. And despite the generally poor health status of bariatric patients prior to surgery, the chance of dying from the operation is exceptionally low.

Even more interesting is that large studies find that the risk of death from any cause is considerably less for bariatric patients over

time than for individuals affected by severe obesity who have never had the surgery. In fact, the data shows up to an 89 percent reduction in mortality, as well as highly significant decreases in mortality rates due to specific diseases. Cancer mortality, for instance, is reduced by 60 percent for bariatric patients. Death associated with diabetes is reduced by more than 90 percent and death from heart disease by more than 50 percent. Also, there are numerous studies that have found improvement or resolution of life-threatening obesity-related diseases following bariatric surgery. According to the ASMBS, the benefits of bariatric surgery, with regard to mortality, far outweigh the risks.

Regardless of health history, getting cut, whether it's on a knee, neck, or belly, does come with some risk. Intubation can cause aspiration, which can lead to pneumonia. You could have an allergic reaction to the anesthesia. The surgeon's knife could slip and—whoops!—give you an extra unexpected slice or two. You could surprise your medical team by bleeding out. A blood clot could develop and travel to your heart, lungs, or brain. Post-bariatric surgery nausea, and pain-pill-induced constipation are common, as are swelling and bruising. The wound site could become infected, or it could be slow to heal. You could get an un-cute scar! And yes, you might die.

This is true for all surgeries, though some are riskier than others. I don't mean to be all doom and gloom, but I'm putting this all out there up front for three reasons:

1. **To be clear about the danger involved in surgery of any kind, including bariatric surgery.** Deciding whether to have bariatric surgery should not be done lightly, and you should always weigh the real risks against the proven outcomes.

2. **To dispel the myth that bariatric surgery is "a quick fix."** For one, bariatric surgery is uncomfortable, if not painful for some, no matter how expert the surgeon. The path to recovery can be challenging as you learn to lead your life in accordance with a lifelong mission of health. To

be successful, you will always have to maintain healthy eating, and just because you'll have a smaller stomach doesn't mean you should just eat smaller portions of Burger King and Snickers bars. Diet and exercise will always be essential components of maintaining weight loss and good health.

3. **To put bariatric surgery in its rightful place among all other surgical medical interventions.** As I said in chapter 4, "Cutting through the Bullshit," no one would give someone a hard time for getting their ACL surgically reconstructed, having a malignancy removed through mastectomy, or undergoing a triple bypass to treat heart disease. Likewise, bariatric surgery is appropriate for the group of people who have a real and serious need (as determined by a medical professional), as it is the *most effective and durable treatment for obesity*. Bariatric surgery results in significant weight loss and aids in the prevention, improvement, and resolution of obesity-related diseases like type 2 diabetes, heart disease, sleep apnea, and some kinds of cancers. It reduces an obese person's risk of premature death by 30 to 40 percent!

Our conversation around bariatric surgery needs to change. We need to accept it as a viable option for a particular population (rough estimates show that as many as *20 million people* in the United States today may qualify and be good candidates for bariatric surgery—yes, you read that correctly: 20 million!). It deserves the same kind of respect we give other forms of life-saving medical treatments. But just as obesity is stigmatized, treatment for obesity is stigmatized too. My own reaction to my sister's suggestion of bariatric surgery is one I now experience on a regular basis, from the other side. As I initially said to my sister, most of us associate this procedure with the super obese. *My 600-Lb. Life*, for example, sends the message that you basically have to be on your deathbed in order for bariatric surgery to be considered. So when I mention bariatric surgery, more often than not, people are shocked, disbelieving, even disgusted. I can see it on their faces. Usually, when I go on to tell them that I've had the surgery and it is one of the best choices I ever made, they try to backpedal, saying things like, "Oh, well, I just mean that I don't like surgery in general" or "Isn't there a better way? That's so extreme" or "I guess that's one way to do it, if you don't want to diet and exercise." They're not wrong about it being extreme, but it is certainly *not* an alternative to maintaining a healthy lifestyle. I always have to bite my tongue, with the knowledge that this is just human nature: we—every single one of us—have gut reactions based on limited or biased information. And just as people have felt free to share their opinions of my body with me, people feel comfortable expressing opinions about a medical procedure they don't know much about.

> So let's get into the guts here!
> What is it? Who is it for?
> How do you get it? How much does it cost?

A note on cost. We will discuss insurance and self-pay options in chapter 8, but as you review the procedure details and the cost ranges in this chapter, I ask that you keep something in mind. Americans generally equate high prices with high quality and low prices with low quality. Much of the time this equation proves to be true, but in researching the costs of bariatric surgery, I have unscientifically found that some of the best surgeons and clinics actually charge the least amount of money. Sometimes a lower cost reflects a business's ability to better manage the costs of goods or services sold. They are able to do this because of years of superior knowledge, relationships in the industry, and high ethical standards (they refuse to offer add-ons or frills that do not actually add any proven value for their customers).

For example, some surgeons doing a gastric sleeve procedure offer a kind of mesh that supposedly helps to close the new stomach lining. It is expensive—around $3,000 extra—and the data does not seem to suggest that it produces many statistically better outcomes than other, much less expensive methods of stapling or suturing. One of the clinics that I explored required me to pay $245 (not covered by insurance) to have an air displacement plethysmography. This involves crawling into a $35,000 egg-shaped chamber (commonly known as a Bod Pod) that measures your weight and volume to determine your body density, then uses this data to calculate your percentage of body fat. While this is likely more accurate than the simple BMI calculation of height and weight, I found it entirely unnecessary and quite claustrophobic. I can certainly see how it might be useful for a professional athlete who needs to intimately understand their body. It could also help to reveal actual body fat for someone who is very muscular and who we otherwise might inaccurately calculate as "overweight" using the simple BMI equation. If this is interesting for you and you want to spend the money, by all means do. For me, I knew that I was fat, my doctor knew I was fat, and I didn't need to go through the rigmarole and spend my time and money on things like this. I needed to save my money for the surgery itself!

Losing Your Gut with Bariatric Surgery

According to the ASMBS, to qualify for bariatric surgery, candidates must

- Have a body mass index of 40 or greater, or be 100 pounds overweight; **or**
- Have a body mass index of at least 35, with related comorbidities such as type 2 diabetes, heart disease, respiratory disorders, osteoarthritis, hypertension, nonalcoholic fatty liver disease, or gastrointestinal disorders; **or**
- *Have a body mass index of at least 30 and other special health conditions,* **and**
- Not have been able to sustain weight loss using other methods.

The last point is very important. No reputable surgeon would perform bariatric surgery on someone who hadn't given conventional weight-loss methods a real and enduring try. Any surgeon worth their salt will ask about your previous weight-loss attempts to determine whether you've exhausted other, less invasive options before they consider you for treatment.

There are three main types of bariatric surgery: gastric sleeve, gastric bypass (Roux-en-Y gastric bypass), and duodenal switch. The fourth type, adjustable gastric band, requires surgery but does not involve any removal or rearrangement of the stomach or intestines. The lesser-known vBloc and gastric balloon, I call "bariatric procedures" because they are less extreme in nature and also don't involve the removal or rearrangement of the stomach or intestines, as you will see. The following information is by no means exhaustive or a substitute for professional medical advice. Rather, I offer it so that you can go into interviews with potential health care providers more prepared. For more information, I recommend the websites of the National Institute of Diabetes and Digestive and Kidney Diseases, the American Society for Metabolic and Bariatric Surgery, and Bariatric Surgery Source. The last website is particularly helpful for digging further into the weeds of insurance coverage.

Gastric Sleeve
(A.K.A. Sleeve, Sleeve Gastrectomy, VSG, LSG)

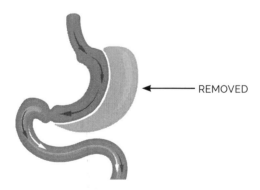

REMOVED

In a gastric sleeve procedure, a surgeon removes up to 80 percent of your stomach, then staples it back together to form a much smaller area—approximately 10 percent of its original size. People love to compare this new shape to a banana or a shirt sleeve. Not only is the area for receiving food smaller, but also it is believed that the partial removal of the stomach affects gut bacteria and ghrelin (a.k.a. ghrr-relin, that mean ol' hunger hormone), changing the patient's appetite and metabolism of food. Gastric sleeve also affects nutrient absorption, so most people have to take a multivitamin for life in order to ensure that their bodies are receiving a healthy amount of nutrients. Short-term studies show that the sleeve is almost as effective as the Roux-en-Y gastric bypass in terms of weight loss and improvement or remission of diabetes. The complication rates of the sleeve fall between those of the adjustable gastric band and the Roux-en-Y gastric bypass.

This is now the most common bariatric surgery (and the one that I had), at approximately 60 percent of all bariatric surgeries performed in 2017. Facts about gastric sleeve surgery:

- It's nonreversible, meaning you'll have a smaller stomach for life.
- It's generally an inpatient procedure, with one to two days of recovery time in the hospital (some patients are eligible for outpatient surgery).
- It's covered by some insurance. Without insurance, the approximate cost of the procedure in 2019 was $19,000. Some surgeons are offering this surgery outpatient (going home same day) with a cost of $12,000. *If I had it to do again, I would choose this option.*
- Within one to three months after, you can eat regular foods (though in much smaller quantities than before surgery).
- People usually have lost 60 to 80 percent of their excess weight by the twelfth month after surgery. At their five-year follow-up, they have generally maintained a loss of 53 to 69 percent of their excess weight.

Gastric Bypass
(A.K.A. Roux-en-Y Gastric Bypass, RYGB)

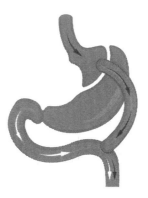

Unlike the gastric sleeve, the gastric bypass does not involve the removal of a portion of your stomach. Instead, the surgeon staples a smaller perimeter (about the size of a walnut) that can hold approximately 1 ounce, or 30 milliliters, then detaches the lower part of the small intestine from your natural stomach and reattaches it to this smaller section. The upper part of the small intestine is then attached to the lower part, so that the digestive enzymes and stomach acid can reach the food once they go through the stomach pouch. The lower section of your stomach and the upper part of the small intestine are still there; they're just being bypassed. This procedure leaves behind only the staples (rather than other foreign devices, like the mesh) and tends to result in similar or slightly more weight loss than the gastric sleeve. But due to the rerouting of the intestines, food will no longer touch a big part of your digestive tract, making it possible that you won't be able to absorb as many vitamins as you might need. Patients who undergo the gastric bypass will need to take a daily multivitamin for life. According to a study published in the October 2013 issue of the *New England Journal of Medicine*, this surgery could increase life expectancy by 89 percent. Facts about the gastric bypass surgery:

- It's still considered by many to be the superior choice of bariatric surgical options in terms of effectiveness.

- It's difficult to reverse due to the rearrangement of organs.
- Five years after, it produces slightly more weight loss than gastric sleeve.
- It's a technically more complex operation than gastric sleeve and has greater complication rates due to more rearrangement of organs.
- It's an inpatient procedure, with two to three days of recovery time in the hospital.
- It's covered by some insurances. Without insurance, the approximate cost of the procedure in 2019 was $24,000.
- You can eat regular foods two to three months after the surgery (though in much smaller quantities than you could before). You will need to watch sugar and fat intake to avoid dumping syndrome. Dumping syndrome occurs when gastric juices and food move from the stomach into the small intestines too quickly, causing cramps, nausea, diarrhea, and vomiting after eating. The risk is higher for patients who have had gastric bypass surgery than patients who have had gastric sleeve surgery. Dietary changes or antidiarrhea medicine may be prescribed to help ease these symptoms.
- People have usually lost 60 to 80 percent of their excess weight by the twelfth month after surgery. At their five-year follow-up, they have generally maintained a loss of 60 to 70 percent of their excess weight.

According to ASMBS, in 2017, gastric sleeve and gastric bypass surgery made up nearly 80 percent of all bariatric surgeries performed in the United States. How much you drink, whether you already suffer from acid reflux, your BMI, and your overall health and risk factors will factor into your and your doctor's decision about which surgery is best for you. In my case, it was clear that sleeve surgery offered me the best mix of risks and rewards.

Duodenal Switch
(A.K.A. Biliopancreatic Diversion)

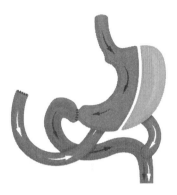

Duodenal switch is something of a combination between the gastric sleeve and the gastric bypass. A surgeon removes approximately 60 to 70 percent of the stomach (like gastric sleeve) and reattaches the small intestine to this smaller stomach pouch (like gastric bypass). Food bypasses through roughly three-quarters of the small intestine, which is reattached below so that enzymes and acids will eventually reach the food. This serves to stop the absorption of fat. Of all the surgeries, duodenal switch is the most complicated and has the highest likelihood of leading to malnourishment in patients afterward. In 2017, this surgery made up less than 1 percent of all bariatric surgeries performed in the United States. Facts about the duodenal switch surgery:

- Of the surgery options, duodenal switch results in the greatest weight loss and is the most effective against diabetes.
- It's nonreversible, meaning you'll have a smaller stomach and rearranged intestines for life.
- Duodenal switch is an inpatient procedure, with two to three days of recovery time in the hospital.
- It's covered by some insurances. Without insurance, the approximate cost of the procedure in 2019 was $27,000.

- You can eat regular foods two to three months after the surgery (though in much smaller quantities than you did before, and you need to watch sugar and fat intake to avoid dumping syndrome).
- People usually improve or even are cured of type 2 diabetes, asthma, hypertension, sleep apnea, and other obesity-related health problems after undergoing this surgery.
- People usually lose 55 to 65 percent of their excess weight after twelve months.
- People have usually have lost 65 to 70 percent of their excess weight at the five-year mark.

Laparoscopic Adjustable Gastric Band
(A.K.A. Band, LAGB, AGB)

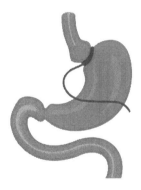

This type of surgery involves a quick (thirty- to sixty-minute) laparoscopic procedure, in which the doctor makes a few small incisions in the upper abdomen, inserts a fiberoptic instrument called a laparoscope and puts a balloon-like silicone band around the top of the stomach. This reduces the size of the stomach pouch itself to approximately an ounce and essentially creates resistance to the natural flow of food, which means you will feel full much more quickly after eating. Digestion occurs normally once food passes through the band, so the risk of nutrient malabsorption is lower in the gastric band procedure than it is in other surgeries. The "adjustable" part of LAGB is maintained through a port (small, round, 25-millimeter silicone implant) just under your belly skin. A tube leads from the port to the band around your stomach. During office visits after surgery, your doctor will use a needle to go through your skin into the port. The more sterile saline solution that's in the band, the tighter the band and the smaller the size of the accessible stomach for food to pass through. In 2017, this surgery made up less than 3 percent of all bariatric surgeries performed in the US. Facts about the laparoscopic adjustable gastric band surgery:

- It's reversible, since organs aren't removed or rerouted.
- It's an inpatient or outpatient procedure. Most patients go home within twenty-four hours of the surgery.
- It's covered by some insurances. Without insurance, the approximate cost of the procedure in 2019 was $15,000.
- It will be six weeks before you can eat regular foods post-surgery (though in much smaller quantities than you could before).
- Foreign objects are left in the body.
- Requires strict adherence to the post-operative diet and to post-operative follow-up visits.
- Highest rate of reoperation.
- Has initially the lowest rate of post-operative complications and mortality, compared with the other bariatric surgeries. However, the risk of complications increases over time (3 to 4 percent a year). Long term, more than a third of patients will experience at least one complication, such as band erosion, band slippage, or port problems.
- People initially lose 20 to 40 percent of excess weight. However, patients are likely to experience significant weight regain and average 15 to 17 percent of excess weight loss at the five-year mark. Over a fourteen-year time period, patients who still had the band in place had lost an average of 15 percent of their excess body weight.

vBloc Therapy

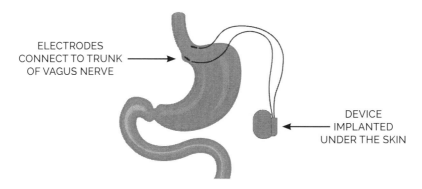

ELECTRODES
CONNECT TO TRUNK
OF VAGUS NERVE

DEVICE
IMPLANTED
UNDER THE SKIN

Vagal Blocking Device Therapy delivers intermittent low-energy, high-frequency electrical pulses to the vagus nerve—which extends from the brain into the digestive tract—to reduce the sensation of hunger. The device, called the Maestro Rechargeable System, includes two electrodes and a rechargeable neuroregulator. It is implanted under the skin below the rib cage through laparoscopic surgery. The device does its thing for approximately twelve hours a day to block hunger and help give the sensation of fullness. Of course, this means you have to wear a device under your skin, and you'll have to charge the lithium battery every other day for roughly thirty minutes. If you don't charge it enough, the device could die and you'd have to go to the doctor to restart it. Facts about the vBloc therapy procedure:

- It's reversible, since organs aren't removed or rerouted. The device can be turned off and removed at any time.
- It's an outpatient procedure. Most patients go home the day of the surgery.
- It's a relatively new surgery and not yet covered by insurance, but the therapy is available for veterans at certain VA hospitals. The approximate cost of the procedure in 2019 was $19,000.
- You can eat regular food immediately after the operation.

- People usually lose an initial 25 to 30 percent of their excess weight and maintain a 20 percent average excess weight loss at the five-year mark.

Gastric Balloon
(A.K.A., Intragastric Balloon)

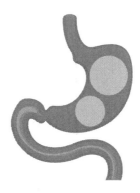

In this procedure, one, two, or three deflated balloons are placed in your stomach via an endoscopic tube that is advanced down the esophagus and into your stomach, then filled with a 650-milliliter saline solution. The balloon or balloons take up space so that you feel full more quickly, which limits how much you can eat. The balloon is left in place for only six months, after which you will have to see your doctor to take it out. This is a short-term and, usually, one-time-only treatment. Facts about the gastric balloon procedure:

- It's reversible, since organs aren't removed or rerouted.
- It's a short outpatient procedure, and most patients go home the day of the procedure.
- Foreign objects are left in the body.
- It's not covered by insurances. The approximate cost of the procedure in 2019 was $8,000.
- You can begin eating regular food at two weeks after the procedure, though you have to be careful of foods like soft bread or pasta that could stick to the balloon.

- People usually lose 20 to 30 percent of their excess weight initially but experience significant regain once the balloons are removed.

The chart on the next two pages shows a quick comparison of some bariatric surgeries/procedures:

Note: The information provided here applies only generally. Patients and procedures may vary depending on individual factors.

Now, I have a strong personal bias about what types of procedures should be considered bariatric *surgery*. I believe that if you don't make profound cuts to the stomach or small intestine, it's not bariatric surgery. If someone qualifies for a surgical intervention because their normal metabolic function is severely compromised, then they need a type of bariatric surgery that addresses the metabolic issue. Bands that are placed around a stomach to restrict food intake do not appear to reconstruct communication between the stomach lining and the brain in the long term. I get concerned when I hear of people spending tens of thousands of dollars on balloons or bands, expecting gastric bypass or sleeve surgery results. Some people have been quite successful with noncutting methods, and certainly there are great reasons not to get cut (one of them being *not getting cut*). But for me, the act of "cutting," while clearly invasive, was the primary point of change.

Of course, the method you choose will not be entirely up to you, and it shouldn't be. Though you may be qualified for surgery (40 BMI, or 30+ BMI with comorbid conditions or other health considerations and a history of failed weight-loss efforts), you will need the help of experts to determine which bariatric surgery, if any, is right for you.

Procedure Name	Gastric Sleeve	Gastric Bypass
Restrictive food intake	X	X
Malabsorption	Limited	X
BMI minimum requirements	30–40% depending on if certain health issues are present	30–40% depending on if certain health issues are present
Percentage of excess weight loss expected after 1 year	60–80% **#1, Year 1**	60–80%
Percentage of excess weight loss and health after 5 years	53–69% Complete resolution or significant improvement for at least 15 obesity-related health conditions, including diabetes, hypertension, and sleep apnea	60–70% Complete resolution or significant improvement for at least 15 obesity-related health conditions, including diabetes, hypertension, and sleep apnea **#1, year 5**
Device or organ remain in body		X
Intestinal reroute		X
Procedure can be performed through laparoscopy	X	X
Time in hospital	1–2 days	1–3 days
Estimated time to return to work	1–2 weeks	1–2 weeks
Brief procedure description	75–90% of patient's stomach is removed, leaving a sleeve-shaped stomach.	Divides the stomach into a small pouch and rearranges the small intestines
Reversible		
Immediate risks* (all procedures may produce nausea and vomiting)	Anesthesia Respiratory Bleeding Blood clots Infection Leaks	Anesthesia Respiratory Bleeding Blood clots Infection Leaks
Long-term risks*	GERD** Stricture Gallbladder	Dumping syndrome Hernia Bowel obstruction Malnutrition/ Iron deficiency Ulcers Stricture Gallbladder Alcoholism

Some risks could lead to serious complications including death (rare).
**gastroesophageal reflux disease*

Duodenal Switch	Adjustable Gastric Band	vBloc	Gastric Balloon
X	X		X
X			
30–40% depending on if certain health issues are present	30% or higher	35% or higher	30% or higher
55–65%	20–40%	25–30%	15–28%
65–70% Is the most effective against diabetes	15–17%	20%	Unknown. Post-balloon removal maintaining weight loss is solely dependent on diet and exercise.
	X	X	X
X			
	X	X	No incision required
1–3 days	1 day	No overnight	Outpatient Nonsurgical
1–2 weeks	1–2 weeks	1–2 days	3–4 days
Combines restriction of sleeved stomach with intestinal bypass	Inflatable band is placed around the top portion of the stomach to restrict food intake.	Implanted device prevents hunger signals from reaching your brain.	Inflated balloon(s) are placed in the stomach.
	Somewhat	X	X
Anesthesia Respiratory Bleeding Blood clots Infection Leaks	Anesthesia Respiratory Bleeding Blood clots Infection	Anesthesia Respiratory Bleeding Blood clots Infection Digestive issues	Sense of heaviness Abdominal or back pain GERD Overinflation
Dumping syndrome Hernia Bowel obstruction Malnutrition/ Iron deficiency Ulcers GERD Stricture Gallbladder Alcoholism	Erosion Food trapping GERD Bowel perforation Ulcers Gallbladder	Neuroregulator malfunction Collapsed lung Interference with other devices Gallbladder	Infection Balloon leak Acute pancreatitis

Trust Your Gut

I spent over a year researching bariatric surgery and interviewing potential surgeons, and I saw the great, the good, the bad (not
in their results but in the way they treated patients), and the sketchy
(just one of those, thankfully). If you have one of the more invasive,
guts-rearranging surgeries, you will be changed for life, so your relationship with your surgeon and medical team will also likely be for life.
Because of this, you need to date around to find someone you trust.
Let me be clear: the vetting process should not be rushed. This book,
along with other reputable resources like the American Society for
Metabolic and Bariatric Surgery website, will assist you on your own
thorough search. Given that I have in-depth, personal experience, I can
offer some red flags for you to look out for.

Bariatric Seminars

Do me the personal favor of avoiding what I call "bariatric cattle calls"
like the plague. Many hospitals, clinics, and surgeons will not see or
talk to you until you have attended one of their seminars. Some of
these are free, while others can cost up to a few hundred dollars, a
fee that will be deducted from the cost of the surgery if you sign up
with them. The two seminars I attended consisted of herding a large
group of fat people into a room with industrial carpeting, bad lighting,
and chairs small enough to be considered torture devices. Everyone sat
around, trying not to make eye contact and appearing generally dazed
and confused. During one of these seminars the presenter talked at us
for forty-five minutes to an hour as the room grew hot and rank. There
was no snack table—because, of course, why would you feed a bunch of
fatties?—and not even some bottled water or stale coffee. The presenter
reeled off stats and facts, using enough jargon and technical language
to make my head spin. "Any questions?" she asked abruptly to signal
the end of her lecture, and then, for the next fifteen minutes or so, one

outspoken person commandeered the Q&A session, while the rest of us sat silent, willing the seminar to just be over.

At the conclusion of these sessions, the cattle lined up to ask the facilitator questions. Many left with those questions unanswered. In her book *Hunger*, Roxane Gay describes her experience at one of these cattle calls, after which she waited a half hour for a one-on-one consultation with the doctor. He flipped through her chart, pronounced her the perfect candidate, and told his intern to schedule her surgery right away, without talking through her options or even looking her in the eye. (Ms. Gay did end up having bariatric surgery, but thankfully not with this doctor!)

I think this practice is deplorable and demeaning. Can you imagine being treated this way if you were diagnosed with brain cancer? Let's extend this fantasy for a moment: imagine that, before a neurosurgeon is willing to see you, you have to sit in an auditorium with a bunch of other people with different kinds of brain cancer and listen to a vague and macrolevel presentation about the possible treatment options and outcomes. That would certainly be more convenient and cost effective for the surgeon or hospital. They could talk to people with astrocytomas, glioblastoma, menigioma, craniopharyngiomas, and lymphomas, all in one fell swoop! But for the patients, this is obviously a big waste of time, not much more helpful than Googling the phrase "brain cancer," which can be done at home, for free, while wearing a bathrobe.

Fortunately, there are more and more bariatric educational videos that you can watch for free online, and I do believe that most medical professionals, given the time, will treat their patients with dignity and respect. If you are not comfortable with the bariatric surgeons closest to you, I recommend you widen your search to outside your own immediate geographical area. Though travel is an added cost, if you can find a better surgeon (or a surgeon you are more comfortable with) who is a plane ride or road trip away, it's well worth the trip. As I've said, this is a medical procedure that you should treat with the upmost seriousness, and in the long run, the cost of some gas or a plane ticket and a hotel room will be nothing compared with the money you'll save with an effective procedure. After my out-of-state bariatric surgery, I have stayed in touch with my surgeon via phone calls and video conference and have visited him in person once when I was nearby on other business.

Endoscopy Debacle

During my presurgery research, I interviewed several post-surgical bariatric patients. One of the patients, Glenn, had originally planned to do the sleeve surgery and had chosen a surgeon out of state from his home in South Carolina. He and his wife flew to meet the surgeon on a Wednesday morning. The surgeon was to perform the presurgical endoscopy that afternoon, in preparation for Glenn's sleeve surgery scheduled the following morning.

One of the common prerequisites for sleeve surgery is an endoscopy. This is an important step that allows your surgeon to make sure you do not have any of the following: hiatal hernia, esophagitis, ulcers, tumors in your upper GI tract, or symptoms of gastroesophageal reflux disease (GERD). Glenn had his endoscopy late Wednesday afternoon, and when he woke up from his procedure, his surgeon had some troubling news. Glenn's results from his endoscopy didn't look good—the endoscopy showed clear signs of asymptomatic GERD. His surgeon told him that he would not be performing the surgery. Glenn had traveled cross-country, followed weeks of the presurgical diet, and completed all the financial and emotional preparations for the surgery. He was devastated.

His surgeon told him that he would be eligible for a gastric bypass but recommended that Glenn go home and spend some time thinking about whether he really wanted this different bariatric surgery. Fortunately, Glenn had already researched the gastric bypass extensively and felt comfortable making an immediate decision to switch surgeries. He had a gastric bypass the next morning. When I first met Glenn, he was several weeks post-surgery and doing really well. I spoke with him nearly two years later, and he was fantastic. He is very happy about how things turned out; for him, a gastric bypass ended up being the right choice.

After talking to Glenn that first time, I decided to get ahead of the endoscopy requirement. As my surgeon was also out of state, I didn't want either to travel there just to get an endoscopy done or to wait (as Glenn did) until right before my scheduled procedure and take my chances on whether it would affect my surgery. So, two and a half months prior to my scheduled surgery date, I called a local gastroenterologist's office to schedule an endoscopy. I was concerned when I was told that the four gastroenterologists in this practice were all scheduling three-plus months out. I hung up and called several other clinics; none could get me in any sooner. I called the original clinic back and asked to be put on a waiting list in the event that there were any cancellations and explained that I had bariatric surgery scheduled in ten weeks and I desperately needed to get in prior. Luckily, the next day they called me and were able to see me for an endoscopy exactly two weeks before my scheduled sleeve surgery. The two procedures were scheduled a little closer together than I would have liked, but I was thankful to get an appointment. I was also overdue for a colonoscopy (because I have celiac, I make sure to get them in the time frames prescribed), and I was able to have that procedure done at the same time.

Three days before my long-awaited endoscopy, the billing office from the gastroenterologist's office called to inform me that my medical insurance had denied coverage for the endoscopy. It would cost me $4,100 out of pocket! I was shocked and panicked. Since my medical insurance wouldn't cover the bariatric surgery, it wouldn't cover any prerequisite procedures either. I lost two days of sleep and made a zillion phone calls to my insurance carrier and the gastroenterologist's office. After two solid days of back and forth, several threats from the gastroenterologist's office that they'd cancel my procedure, and finally, direct help from the very kind gastroenterologist, my insurance company agreed to cover the procedure based on needing an endoscopy for ongoing symptoms related to my previously diagnosed celiac disease. It was perhaps the only time I have ever been glad that I have celiac!

If you are planning to self-pay for bariatric surgery and have a condition for which you may need an endoscopy (besides your upcoming surgery)—GERD, difficulty swallowing, upper abdominal pain,
or celiac disease—be sure that you see a gastroenterologist about
your other condition in addition to your upcoming bariatric surgery.
Otherwise, you may be looking at an additional bill for the endoscopy,
as I was.

Unnecessary Tests or Procedures

A few of the bariatric surgeons I interviewed required a sleep apnea
study. This makes sense, as sleep apnea is common among people who
are obese. This condition's most famous symptoms are snoring and the
kind of choking, gasping, and pauses in breathing that will scare the
bejeezus out of the person who is sharing your bed. If left untreated,
sleep apnea can cause serious health issues, including high blood pressure, heart conditions, liver problems, type 2 diabetes, stroke, and even
death. A bariatric surgery patient who has sleep apnea must treat the
condition with a CPAP machine before and for several months following the procedure, to reduce risk of surgical complications both during
and after surgery.

Having said this, I found the sleep study one-size-fits-all mandate
to be frustrating, because not all obese people have apnea; in fact, many
do not. There are plenty of thin folks who have it, like my husband who,
at 6 feet 1 and 175 pounds (BMI 20), suffers from sleep apnea that is
caused by some esophageal issues. Because of this, we are a family with
apnea awareness, and I have asked him many times over the years if I
snore. He has reported that, other than occasionally lightly snoring
when I first drift off to la-la land or when I have a cold, I do not. And I
show no other telltale signs of sleep apnea, such as morning headaches,
daytime sleepiness, lack of concentration, poor memory, or irritability.
When I shared this information with a bariatric doctor who initially
demanded that I participate in a full-blown sleep apnea study, he was
skeptical. He and I negotiated and agreed that I would wear a fingertip

monitor (a small clip-like device that fits over the tip of the finger) to do an overnight oxygen-saturation-level test instead. This test can rapidly detect even small changes in how efficiently oxygen is being carried through your blood to the extremities farthest from the heart. If the results concerned him, then I would agree to submit to the sleep apnea study.

I wore that monitor for a couple nights, barely getting any sleep because I was too worried it might fall off. Three days after returning the "little black data box," a nurse called to give me the results. My average oxygen level had been at 99 percent, she told me, but had dropped to 93 percent six or seven times throughout each night. "Wonderful!" I said. "Looks like I won't need to do the full-blown sleep apnea study."

"Actually, if your oxygenation levels fall more than five points more than five times during the night, it indicates sleep apnea," she said. She told me that I was now required to participate in the full sleep study. She went on to say that if they did indeed find (based on the full sleep study) that I have sleep apnea—and she guessed they would, as almost everyone that comes to their clinic for bariatric surgery is diagnosed with sleep apnea—then I would be required to get a CPAP machine and wear it for at least four hours a day for thirty days prior to the surgery. She further explained that they put a monitor on the machine that would clock how much time I'd spent using it. If I failed to meet their time requirement, I would not be eligible for surgery until I did. She also let me know that they have strict requirements regarding the machine immediately post-surgery during my recovery in the hospital. She closed the discussion by telling me that she was aware that their patients absolutely hate this mandate. When they are hurting and vomiting from nausea after the surgery and are forced to wear the machine, it often makes them feel like they are suffocating!

Now, don't get me wrong. As a rule, I am a dream patient, compliant and obedient, following doctors' advice to a T. I'm not shy about or resistant to obtaining a proper diagnosis and treatment plan, even if it means I have to overhaul my life. But in this instance, something just didn't feel right. I didn't have any symptoms of sleep apnea, and having seen firsthand the struggles my husband has gone through using a CPAP machine, I didn't love the idea of having to use one if it wasn't totally necessary. And it seemed odd to me that nearly *every* patient who came into their clinic was positively diagnosed. After a little research, I realized that if I used my insurance to pay for the sleep study (which, by the way, the bariatric clinic itself would perform), the results would go on my permanent medical record, potentially affecting life insurance and other considerations for the rest of my natural-born life! If I chose not to run it through my insurance, it would cost me $3,000 out of pocket. Then the punchline came—if they diagnosed me with sleep apnea, I would be required to rent a machine (you guessed it: from them) for $300.00 a month for a minimum of four to six months.

I weighed my options. Then I said, "Thanks, but no thanks!"

The clinic called me back a week later to tell me that the surgeon had decided to "be very nice" and waive the "sleep study thing." And he'd agreed to perform the surgery right away! Did I want to go ahead and schedule it?

Needless to say, I did not move forward with this clinic. I later found out that they just so happened to be running a large sleep study at the time I was looking into them, and they were gathering as many test subjects as they could get. What a coincidence. (This was the sketchy clinic I mentioned.)

NOTE: It is common for bariatric clinics to require sleep studies for patients who intend to use insurance. This is particularly important if a patient's BMI is less than 40 and the surgeon is trying to help the patient qualify for insurance coverage by legitimately substantiating this morbid condition, if it exists. So, if you show the telltale signs of having sleep apnea and you are trying to qualify for insurance coverage for bariatric surgery, then keep an open mind about participating in a sleep study—it can save your life and your pocketbook! However, if you were like me—self-pay and no symptoms—be cautious, as sleep apnea can turn into a costly and arduous diagnosis, and the diagnosis may not always be 100 percent trustworthy.

Cavalier Attitudes about GERD

Gastroesophageal reflux disease (GERD) is a fancy way to say heartburn. It is caused by stomach acid moving up into the esophagus, often due to weakness of or a tear in the hiatus, a small opening in the diaphragm that connects the esophagus and the stomach. GERD can be really painful and, if frequent, very disruptive to the sufferer's life. Besides heartburn, people with GERD may also experience nausea, a burning sensation in the throat, a bitter taste in the mouth, chest discomfort, bloating, and dry mouth. Often obese people already suffer from GERD; according to the Obesity Action Coalition, people with a BMI of 30 or higher are two and a half times more likely than people with a BMI under 25 to have it. Bariatric surgery can make the symptoms of GERD better. It can also make them worse.

Many of the bariatric surgeons that I spoke with had an attitude of "Yep, you'll probably suffer from long-term acid reflux post-surgery. Just a fact of life." Without batting an eyelash, one doctor told me it could feel like having a heart attack every single day.

It's one thing to be honest about potential side effects; it's another to be cavalier when it comes to pain. Yes, you could have GERD after surgery. But a good surgeon will promise to do their best to manage this if it does come to pass. This willingness was at the top of my priority list when vetting surgeons, and the surgeon I ultimately chose talked to me in depth about how his surgical technique helped patients avoid GERD. He told me that his goal is to make life better, not worse, for his patients, and having severe GERD and being on lifelong prescriptions to try to minimize the symptoms does not make life better. The incidence of GERD in his patients was drastically lower than the national average.

Be sure to have this conversation, and if a surgeon or anyone on the medical team shrugs you off or seems resigned to your having GERD long term, that is not the right clinic for you.

NOTE: Prior to sleeve surgery I never had any acid reflux symptoms. For three months post-surgery, I did have some mild GERD and took a daily pill to combat the symptoms. After my new small stomach learned that it no longer needed to produce stomach acid at the same rate it did presurgery, I have not had any further issues.

Cutting to the Chase

Come prepared with a list of questions to ask a potential surgeon. Even if you think you know what type of bariatric surgery you need, it's important that you do your due diligence and ask at least some basic questions about the surgeon and the surgery. Here are some ideas:

- Am I a candidate for weight-loss surgery? Why or why not?
- What type of bariatric surgery is best for me? Why?
- Are you a licensed physician and board certified in obesity medicine?
- What is your philosophy on weight gain? (You want to know if they acknowledge that obesity is a metabolic rather than a moral disease.)
- How much weight can I expect to lose?
- How many surgeries have you performed?
- What surgeries do you perform?
- How do you keep costs low for your patients while ensuring they receive the highest-quality care?
- (Dependent on the bariatric surgery) What are your incident rates of post-surgery complications (both short and long term) for things like GERD, strictures, leaks, and bowel obstruction among your patients?
- What is the patient death rate from bariatric surgery in your practice? And for the bariatric surgeries that you have performed? What caused the deaths in each of these circumstances?

- What kind of presurgery testing and dieting do you require?
- What kind of care do you offer after the surgery? How long do you expect the recovery to take?
- What is the post-surgery diet?
- How available are you to help after the bariatric surgery if a concern arises?
- What are my next steps?

CHAPTER 7

Clear-Cut

*The best time to plant a tree was 20 years
ago. The second-best time is now.*
—Chinese proverb

I interviewed and researched dozens of doctors, and while they all had similar medical guidelines to follow, each seemed to have their own unique approach when it came to surgical approval and qualification criteria, presurgery testing, presurgery diet, surgical setting, length of hospital stay, pain medication, post-surgery diet, and required follow-up.

I spent months searching for the right doctor, but somehow I kept coming up short. As I continuously learned more about bariatric surgery and my own surgical needs and wants, I realized that I still hadn't met someone with whom I felt completely safe and respected. When I started out looking for a bariatric surgeon, my most important criteria in choosing someone were surgical skill and safety metrics. Thankfully, surgeons who perform more than one hundred bariatric procedures per year tend to have an excellent safety record, and in general, there is very little variation in the safety records of the vast majority of bar-iatric surgeons in the US. Because most of them are able to perform these surgeries so safely, I found that I had the opportunity to select a surgeon based on other, more personal factors.

Finally, after nearly a year of searching, I finally found the One. The first thing I liked about him was that he didn't seem to be trying to make a sale, or to get me in and out the door as quickly as possible. The office staff was friendly and competent. No one seemed to have an agenda beyond helping the patients figure out the option that would be right for them. In fact, Dr. Matthew Weiner told me early on that if I decided to be his patient, he would be one of my primary doctors for life, so I'd better be sure that I both trusted and liked him before sign-ing on. We spent a significant amount of time discussing my surgical options, what the surgery itself would entail (blood, guts, and all), and the associated risks. He had a good treatment strategy that was far-sighted and practical, as well as a reasonable recommended presurgery diet. He seemed to make a great effort to stay connected to the bariat-ric community and offered a ton of educational resources through his weight-loss program: A Pound of Cure. Dr. W also routinely performed multiple different types of bariatric surgery, which was very important to me as I knew he was skilled and knowledgeable in many areas. His both deep and broad expertise assured me that he was offering me the best surgery for my individual needs rather than steering me toward the surgery that was most convenient for him.

The surgery would be performed in a hospital, not a clinic, in case of emergency, and the anesthesiologist my surgeon partnered with specialized in working with obese patients. Preparations included a comprehensive regimen to avoid nausea and vomiting post-surgery, an essential when you have stitches in your belly, and a plan for getting off painkillers within a couple days. Dr. W's post-op diet was very differ-ent from most that I'd reviewed. His philosophy was that the patient should get back on real food quickly to ensure proper intake of micro-nutrients, instead of relying on highly processed protein shakes.

All in all, he was the perfect choice: knowledgeable and able to translate that knowledge for the layperson, empathetic, and professional in every way. Plus he had a great sense of humor and was willing to have the long, hard conversations with me about my fears and expectations. Never did I feel he was judging me or looking down on me—he was clear in his firm belief that obesity is a real disease that warrants real medical treatment. Most important of all, he was an animal lover. Well, OK, maybe not the most important criterion, but it is important!

What mattered more to me was that he did not try to sugarcoat anything. He was very open about the statistical outcomes of the surgeries that he had performed (not all bariatric surgeons are so forthright about their success and less-than-success rates). His were some of the best numbers that I had seen, especially those related to gastroesophageal reflux disease. He never promised me a quick fix or told me that the road post-surgery would be paved in gold. "It won't be easy," he said, "but I think you can do it."

Prepping the Gut to Be Cut: The Presurgery Diet

One thing that I liked about Dr. W's approach was his preoperative diet. The pre-op diet is a requirement for all cut-gutting bariatric surgeries and is designed for fast and short-term weight loss that is not meant to be maintained over the long run. Losing weight quickly depletes the liver of fat and glycogen, making the surgery easier to perform.

Dr. W explained that the most effective way to lose weight quickly is by severely restricting calorie intake. The preoperative diet I followed required me to limit my calorie intake to around 800 calories per day with very few carbohydrates. He told me that men, high-BMI patients, people with diabetes, and those whose weight is concentrated in their belly are more difficult to operate on. Some people who fell into those categories were required to follow the preoperative diet for two to four weeks, as a critical component to a safe surgery. I was fortunate to only have to follow it for one week.

Some presurgical patients are required to follow an all-liquid protein shake diet, with no "chewable food." Dr. W. recommended using meal-replacement protein shakes that contained 15 to 20 grams of protein, less than 3 grams of sugar, and less than 200 calories each. He also allowed unlimited green vegetables and unlimited use of seasonings and spices as well as unlimited calorie-free drinks (anything less than 10 calories per serving) on the preoperative diet (artificial sweeteners were discouraged post-op). Oils, butter, and avocados were verboten.

Below is the presurgical diet I followed.

All women with a BMI <50

- Two protein shakes every day (one for breakfast, one for lunch)
- A healthy, low-carbohydrate dinner (<400 calories)
- Unlimited calorie-free liquids
- Unlimited green vegetables
- Start one week prior to your surgical date.

All men and women with a BMI >50
(the diet is the same but twice as long in duration)

- Four protein shakes every day
- Unlimited calorie-free liquids
- Unlimited green vegetables
- Start two weeks prior to your surgical date (or longer if instructed).

The preoperative diet was difficult to follow, and I was thankful it was only a short-term program. I got through it by telling myself that (1) it was the very last "diet" I would ever follow, and (2) it was important to have my liver and abdomen in the best condition possible for surgical safety. Every time I thought about cheating, I recalled these two facts. I knew I would blame myself if anything went wrong and I hadn't done exactly what I was supposed to presurgery.

A Gut-Punching Breakup

I believe there are generally two types of people when it comes to eating preferences: those (like me) who eat "regular" food only as a means to an end—the end being DESSERT; and those like my barbequing DietDisser neighbor Anthony, who could go a whole year without eating a piece of cake or a candy bar and never even miss it. Anthony is all about savory and salty food and *way* too much of it! If you are very unlucky, you have both propensities: a sugar and savory food inclination.

A couple weeks before beginning my preoperative diet, I forced myself to deeply reflect on my eating habits and was painfully honest with myself about what changes I would need to make in my diet and behaviors post-bariatric surgery. Ultimately, I decided to sit down with a pen and paper (old school) and write a "breakup" letter with sugar.

I'll admit, I've had some experience in my life with breakups, both as the breakupee and as the breaker-uper. Some have been more painful than others, but this one was in the top five of zingers! While I do recognize that writing a breakup letter with sugar is weird, and perhaps a bit tragic, it was a necessary part of my process:

Dear Sugar,

It seems surreal to be writing you this letter, not only because, well, let's face it, it is a strange thing to do-write a letter to a sweet, white substance-but also because, until recently, I didn't fully recognize the full extent to which you have been a part of my life. You are a being, an entity, something/someone I have interacted with daily, sometimes hourly. I sought you out at every turn, missed you when we hadn't seen each other for even a brief time, and was euphoric each time we connected.

With the exception of my parents, I have had the longest relationship of my life with YOU, nearly fifty years! And unlike my sweet parents (no pun intended), you have been with me, literally part of me, almost every day. You have had a front-row seat to my every waking (and sleeping) thought, my feelings and interactions with the world. In truth, I now realize you have been my best friend since I began eating solid foods. There are so many things I have grown to love about you over our half century together:

- Your availability—you are everywhere.
- Your diversity—I never tire of you. You come in all shapes, sizes, colors, levels of sweetness, consistencies, and temperatures; you can be expensive, cheap, unique, or common. You are the truest art form I have ever known.
- When I am happy, you explode in my body and make me happier.
- When I am bored, you entertain me.
- When I am stressed, I rush to find you somewhere/anywhere, just even a little bit of you, and you calm me.
- When I am sad, your taste is flat, but your effects are gently powerful, returning me to a sense of normalcy.
- You give me "sugasms."

In my early childhood, you were a reward. I received you when I had behaved well or when I was hurt. I found you in the form of Lucky Charms, red licorice, yum-yum cookies, Twinkies, chocolate cake, Dip-a-Stick, Big Hunk, Mountain candy bars, Lemonheads, Zotts, Pop Rocks, and A&W Rootbeer floats (to name a few of my favorites). In my insecure and tumultuous teens, I sought you everywhere: my other best friend Teri and I would walk for miles to the local 7-Eleven to purchase all the candy that our allowances would afford us. When I could drive, I made sure to find you every morning on a secret detour to the doughnut shop before school, during school in the vending machines, and in the evenings (either at home or away). You were one of my greatest passions growing up, and looking back, I spent a lot of time seeking you out alone (or with others). You never let me down.

In recent times, I have pondered at length why you were such a huge part of my early years (one to eighteen years old). After I turned over every rock of blame and shame, I recognized, you were just there—that's it. Like the lifelong friend that you first happen to meet in 1977 in a record store—they were there, you were there, and the rest is history. You and I had a fine relationship (or so I thought) during my youth, but by the time I reached adolescence, my parents didn't seem too keen on your presence. Thankfully, I was clever and hid you reasonably well. Never once did I think about giving you up, and never did I think about what our relationship may mean or why I was obsessed with you.

Now at nearly fifty years old, I have spent decades pushing you away only to have you reappear over and over again. By now, the extra 80 pounds that I am carrying are the least of my problems! I have high blood pressure, urine that smells like a box of Cheerios, fatty liver, kidneys and a heart that are not working optimally, and a whole host of other physical ailments that I know you have brought upon me. Most devastating is that I fear early mortality and type 2 diabetes because of you. In the end, you are killing me and, in that slow death process, everything I used to love about myself.

So, dear Sugar, I am breaking up with you forever. You have been my longest friend, and for the good years and times I am very thankful. However, if I had it all to do again, I would give up all of our times together, every last one of them, because you have never really been my friend; in fact, you have been a slow poison, a killer. Your intentions were always bad. I should have seen this long ago, but as they say, love is blind and the power of denial strong. Your pleasure is ephemeral and your wreckage lasting. As Tom Petty said, "Don't come around here no more. You darken my door." It is irreconcilable, finished, over, and nonnegotiable. The end!

Looking back at my breakup letter, I remember feeling a sinking dread when I wrote it. At the time, I imagined I would feel a pit in my stomach for a long time over parting ways with sugar. However, post-surgery, my hormones and chemical brain impulses have changed significantly. The feeling of devastating loss was quickly replaced by a profound feeling of relief—of being free from a chemical feedback loop that had once driven me uncontrollably. With forty-nine years of ingrained eating behavior under my belt, I do have to remind myself at times to continue to make the right food choices in varying situations, but my healthy eating habits and daily food choices are now well established. The urge to eat sugary sweets is a fleeting thought these days.

Gut Check:
The One-Chance Factor

My mom used to tell me that there are only two things that are certain in life: death and taxes. Outside of these two (and maybe even these are negotiable, depending on what you believe about an afterlife or reincarnation, or how much jail time you are willing to serve), the world is full of possibilities. As a hopeless romantic and a glass-is-half-full kind of person, I find myself believing this to be true. Life, however, has reminded me on occasion that all doors don't remain open forever.

I was surprised to learn that one of the leading reasons that qualified candidates for bariatric surgery don't move forward is fear based on the "one chance" factor. You can go to rehab multiple times for addiction issues with sex, drugs, or alcohol, but food is its own unique beast. Unlike an alcoholic, who can stop drinking, you can't just stop eating. And you cannot (usually) get bariatric surgery multiple times to lose the desired weight. If you've had a big part of your stomach removed or your guts rearranged, there's limited next steps. The fact that we're given only one shot stops many people in their tracks. It's like Olympic athletes who get only one shot their entire lives in front of the camera at their chosen sport.

To get a better grasp on this "onetime" bariatric surgery preparation, consider this question: what have you done to prepare for a simple
run-of-the-mill diet in the past? I have waited to start it until I had
communicated with and gotten the support of everyone living under
the same roof as me, got my workout clothes and kitchen equipment
all sorted out and ready to go, and identified a specific exercise routine along with the dietary restrictions and recommendations. Then
I'd choose X date and X time to begin, a moment heavy (pun intended)
with significance. I'd meticulously prepare a shopping list, buy grocer-
ies, and get to work making precooked meals. As if all of this logistical
prep wasn't enough, I also required myself to be in the right emotional,
mental, and physical state before I could begin. Was I calm yet excited
and confident? Did I have enough energy, and was my immune system
strong? Was the plan well considered and complete from start to finish? Basically, I overthought everything. (Even with all this intensive
prep, there were a few times that, in the end, I just wasn't feeling it,
and I ended up throwing away most of the specialty or meticulously
prepared food.) As I've mentioned, usually all my good intentions were
for naught, and I'd lose a few pounds, only to gain it back again. I'd
get discouraged, not to mention hungry, tired, and irritable, and so I'd
quit. Then time would pass, I'd forget the frustration and futility of the
last attempt, and I'd do it all over again. I don't believe I am alone in
all of this fuss over diets, which I could usually follow for only a couple
weeks, or a couple months, tops! Think about it: if this is how much
emotional and logistical energy we put into dieting, then imagine what
it takes to prepare for bariatric surgery.

The bariatric surgeons I talked to around the US told me that the
average time it takes someone to have bariatric surgery from the day
they begin to consider it is seven months. Interestingly, if a person
goes beyond 1.4 years without having the surgery, it becomes much
less likely that they will ever head under the knife as time goes on. For
some, reasons such as lack of money or family support pale in comparison to the fear that if this one chance doesn't work, nothing will, and
If I fail, I'm screwed.

There is no doubt that this concern is valid. While a surgeon will tell you there are revision surgeries available depending on what type of bariatric surgery you have, it is not something most people want to undergo more than once in their life. Therefore, it is very important to be absolutely ready and make the absolute most of the surgery. So, yes, you must be mindful of the once-in-a-lifetime seriousness of bariatric surgery *and* you must also not let that paralyze you.

Cutting Teeth:
Phases of Bariatric Surgery

Phases of bariatric surgery:

- Phase 1: Infancy—The Long-Term Weight Struggle
- Phase 2: Toddler—Starting to Swim: Considering and Preparing for Bariatric Surgery
- Phase 3: Jumping In—Surgery
- Phase 4: Floaties—Recovering from Surgery
- Phase 5: The Lazy River—Significant Weight Loss
- Phase 6: Open Water—Sustainable Weight Loss

Phase 1:
Infancy, The Long-Term Weight Struggle

Human babies are some of the most helpless and vulnerable creatures on earth. Defenseless. This is how I often felt when I was overweight and struggling with food, health, and society's judgment. Much of the time I felt powerless over the scale and dependent on the help of others for change. My long-term struggle to learn and thrive as a healthy human is in many ways like being an infant.

Phase 2:
Toddler—Starting to Swim: Considering
and Preparing for Bariatric Surgery

When I was a toddler, it was important to my parents that they teach me how to swim. Their first step was to get me used to and comfortable in the water: my parents took me to a local pool and held me close while they twirled me around and I explored this new environment.

During phase 2 of bariatric surgery, you are twirling around in a flurry of activity as you interview surgeons and find the "One" for you, and get used to the idea of having surgery. You are exploring this new environment and deciding whether you are willing to learn how to swim. You are also figuring out how you are going to pay for the surgery (and related expenses). Any swimming instructor will tell you that this is one of (if not *the*) most important phases. If this goes badly, all bets may be off! Be patient and try to keep a positive attitude. During this phase, you will also be participating in your presurgical appointments with the nutritionist (and others) and doing the beginning work on changing your eating habits and lifestyle to set yourself up for long-term success post-surgery.

As a notorious planner, I got ready for both the worst-case scenarios *and* what life after surgery would mostly likely look like (at least what I could envision at the time). The following is a checklist of these extra to-do items:

- Update living will.
- Write notes to my loved ones.
- Apply for Family Medical Leave Act (FMLA) for time off from work.
- Exercise to be stronger for surgery.
- Pack according to hospital pack list from surgeon, for example, comfortable clothing to wear in the hospital and for travel home.

Phase 3:
Jumping In—Surgery

After several trips to the pool, I came to trust my parents with "life and limb," and so when my dad suggested I jump off the side of the pool into his arms (and followed up with some gentle encouragement), I agreed. Surgery is a bit like jumping off the side of the pool into your surgeon's arms. You must trust that the surgeon will do everything in their power to keep you safe and vastly improve your life.

Of all of the phases, this is probably the most feared. It is also the easiest. The morning of my surgery, I showed up at the hospital early. They verified that I had followed my presurgical diet. I dressed in the glamorous hospital gown, and they set up the equipment to monitor my heart rate and blood pressure and placed the IV. I tried to stay calm, thank the medical assistants and nurses that were prepping me, and visualized waking up with a new set point. My type A personality has a serious problem with not being in control at all times (although I do realize that being in control is just an illusion), but I had already told myself to sit back, breathe, let go, manifest positive thoughts into the universe, and trust.

The brief time that I spent in the hospital was a bit of a blur. I do not remember feeling much pain or being at all nauseated after the procedure. I was determined to drink water and get up and walk around as soon as my doctor told me I was able. Thankfully, all went according to plan, and I was into the next phase within a couple days.

Phase 4:
Floaties—Recovering from Surgery

After my parents helped me acclimate to the swimming pool and helped me see that it was more likely that swimming would be a fun and positive experience rather than a drowning event, it was time for me to take a new step forward. Remember the goal here was not that I just show up willingly in the pool splashing around and jumping into my father's arms; it was to swim independently and confidently in all kinds of waters and conditions. In this phase of learning to swim, I graduated from being in the pool in my parents' arms to wearing floaties, little inflatable arm swim aids designed to help the wearer float in the water. This transition was riddled with anxiety. The helplessness was gone, but being let go in the water was an unfamiliar change that brought about new hopes and new dangers. Thank goodness, my parents were still very close by.

Phase 4 is about basic survival. You will be forced to pay very close attention to every single bite of food you put in your mouth. Your mind and activities will be heavily focused on doing the "right" things and making sure you are hydrated every day. Remember your body *finally* realizes it is *way* overfed. Before surgery my body and mind were constantly pushing me to act out behaviors that helped ensure I would remain at my high set point weight. Pre-surgery if I deviated from my set point through not eating enough, I would feel dizzy, low energy, and "hangry" (hungry and angry). In phase 4, my body finally realized it had plenty of fat storage. Not eating much wasn't a challenge, and I actually had significantly increased energy and mental capacity. Your doctor (like my parents) will stay very near you and help you navigate these first baby steps into your newfound independence—listen to him or her! My doctor says this phase is a temporary gift: the hunger and cravings are gone, giving you a unique opportunity to change to a healthier diet. After your incisions heal, you can even start exercising. The pounds seem to fly off, and this stage is quite exhilarating. However, if you fight this opportunity and try to get back to your old eating habits (just in much smaller portions), at the very least you will make yourself sick, or, much worse, you will eventually experience weight gain. By the end of this phase, you will have lost all or almost all of your excess weight.

Phase 5:
The Lazy River—Significant Weight Loss

When I was strong enough in the pool and could coordinate my kicking, breathing, and arm movements, the floaties were removed and I was left to swim on my own from one side of the pool to the other. My parents remained in the pool area but moved farther away. This phase of swimming in the pool with supervision, but without direct and continuous monitoring, lasted for several years. As I became a stronger swimmer, I also learned how to dive, float, and perform a variety of different strokes. With each new technique I learned, I felt more in control and better able to save myself should something go wrong.

Phase 5 will last anywhere from eighteen months to five years, depending on individual factors as well as the type of surgery. The surgery and all of its miracle mechanisms are working at their peak now, and you will wonder if your old weight-loss struggles were just a bad nightmare. Your food intake will still be restricted, and some old unhealthy foods may still not agree with you. If you listen, your body and mind will steer you strongly toward being active and eating healthy whole foods, and you will have much better appetite control. You will feel strong and empowered to make good choices. However, during this phase you can divert to old bad habits if you're not careful. My doctor calls this "head hunger." You *think* you are hungry for a cheeseburger and fries, but that thinking is an old behavior pattern begging to be played out again, not a *real* food craving. It is relativity easy at this stage to recognize this and quickly move on to a chicken salad instead. By doing so, not only will you maintain your health and weight, but also you won't take unwanted and unpleasant trips to the restroom. During this phase, it is critical for you to demonstrate that you have the ability and desire to recognize old bad behaviors and continue with your mindful eating strategies.

Phase 6:
Open Water—Sustainable Weight Loss

After several years of swimming in a temperature-controlled pool that was cleaned and sanitized regularly, and having the support of lifeguards all around me in case I found myself in trouble, I took the next big step in my swimming evolution and obtained both my lifeguard certification and my scuba certification. Not only did I find myself now swimming in the open ocean full of unpredictability, but also I no longer had the crutches around me that I had come to take for granted. In fact, in becoming a lifeguard, I *was* the crutch!

It is helpful to understand that this last phase is a natural and predictable outcome of bariatric surgery. My doctor advised me early on that eventually most weight-loss surgery patients experience a return in their appetite, food cravings, and lack of enthusiasm for exercise. Unfortunately, as my mother always said, "all good things in life must come to an end." But this ending, thank goodness, doesn't usually mean a return to where you were presurgery.

Why does this happen? It is important to know that when or if it does, you have done nothing wrong, and your surgeon hasn't either. And many of the explanations you'll find on the internet are wholly untrue. Despite what Google tells you, your stomach has not stretched out again (multiple endoscopy tests on bariatric surgery patients have revealed that this is a falsehood).

I believe the explanation is simple: our bodies have healed (just maybe a little too well). I am squarely in this phase now, and I am happy to report that I am successfully swimming in open waters. To date, I have been up and down a maximum of 3 pounds after hitting my new set point. I work at it, every day. Previously, I had developed a lifetime of bad habits, and it will take me another lifetime to eradicate them. The vast difference now is that post-surgery, if I deviate, I get myself back on course—immediately! My body is my friend now. It is responsive and cooperative, and we work together to maintain mindful eating and health. This dynamic was unthinkable to me presurgery.

My body was more like a toddler throwing a temper tantrum at the side of the pool because she doesn't want to learn how to swim.

According to the American Society for Metabolic and Bariatric Surgery, "As many as 50 percent of patients may regain a small amount of weight (approximately 5 percent) two years or more following their surgery. However, longitudinal studies find that most bariatric surgery patients maintain successful weight-loss long-term. . . . Such massive and sustained weight reduction with surgery is in sharp contrast to the experience most patients have previously had with non-surgical therapies."

CHAPTER 8

Cutting through the Red Tape

Courage is being scared to death
but saddling up anyway.
—John Wayne

Cutting through
Insurance and Self-Pay

For better or worse (mostly worse), you'll have plenty of time to practice mindfulness while getting your finances in order. Some bariatric surgeries are supposedly covered by regular medical insurance,
Medicaid, Medicare, or the Affordable Care Act. Still, when it comes
to covering the procedure, insurance companies would rather cut their
nose off to spite their face. Many won't pay the $12,000 to $35,000
for bariatric surgery; they would rather pay hundreds of thousands of
dollars for obesity-related disease, illnesses, and treatments, such as

triple-bypass surgery after a heart attack, hospital stays after a stroke, a CPAP machine for sleep apnea, insulin to treat diabetes, and prescription blood pressure pills—the list goes on and on. An article published by the American Society for Metabolic and Bariatric Surgery says it best:

> Despite the overwhelming high quality data demonstrating the safety and benefits of metabolic and bariatric surgery, universal insurance coverage for treatment of clinically severe obesity has not been established, unlike for other potentially life-threatening diseases such as cancer, heart disease, and diabetes (for which obesity is a powerful risk factor). Furthermore, unlike coverage for patients with other life-threatening diseases, those with clinically severe obesity often face a myriad of arbitrarily imposed criteria to obtain insurance authorization for metabolic and bariatric surgery, which includes documentation of supervised diet attempts of various lengths of time (e.g., typically 3–18 months), with specified providers and formats. . . . [These diets] must also meet a specified percentage of preoperative weight loss of 5–15%. . . . Insurance-mandated preoperative weight loss requirements are strictly enforced without consideration of the severity of obesity present; the status of other life-threatening co-morbid conditions or life circumstances that may force a patient to miss a required visit; or whether the patient can afford the additional costs of the adjunct dietary and exercise programs, medications, and visits to providers to comply with the requirements.
>
> The outcome of insurance-mandated preoperative weight loss requirements is patient attrition, delay in obesity treatment, progression of obesity and

associated life-threatening co-morbid conditions, and increased direct and indirect health care costs.

A National Institutes of Health (NIH) consensus statement does not recommend weight loss before surgery, understanding that the majority of individuals with clinically severe obesity have suffered a lifelong battle with obesity and have almost uniformly failed multiple prior efforts without long-term efficacy. The provider, the statement says, should be able to determine what constitutes failed efforts for each patient. The majority of patients who are denied insurance coverage for bariatric surgery and cannot afford to pay for it out of pocket will experience progression of their obesity and obesity-related comorbid conditions, particularly diabetes, as well as a higher incidence of new-onset diabetes, hypertension, and sleep apnea while awaiting insurance approval, even though it is well understood that the likelihood of achieving healthy weight without surgery is exceedingly low. I don't take this to mean that NIH does not support bariatric surgeons putting their patients on a short preoperative diet in order to get the abdomen ready for surgery whereby lowering surgical risk. Instead, I believe the NIH is saying that insurance companies and doctors should not continue to unnecessarily require obese patients to diet for three to eighteen months (whereby postponing surgery and potentially making them sicker) just to prove one last time that a diet will fail them. Another not-so-fun aspect of these lengthy insurance dieting prerequisites is that if the patient loses too much weight, they suddenly won't qualify for the surgery. That would be great if most people then kept the weight off. But I know all too well that the minute the unrealistic diet stops, the weight gloms back on with a vengeance! What is a person that needs bariatric surgery and wants insurance to cover it to do? To me, this practice borders on unethical.

We know that the odds are very low that a morbidly obese person will achieve a healthy weight within a twelve-month period of time without bariatric surgery. A longitudinal study recently published by the United Kingdom's Clinical Practice Research Datalink followed, over a period of nine years, 76,704 obese men and 99,791 obese women who had not undergone bariatric surgery. The study found that the annual probability of a morbidly obese person attaining normal weight was 1 in 1,290 for men and 1 in 677 for women. The ASMBS says: "Patients seeking surgical treatment for clinically severe obesity should therefore be evaluated for eligibility based on their initial pre-senting BMI and not be penalized or denied care for weight lost as part of insurance-mandated preoperative weight loss."

I can't delineate a one-size-fits-all list of steps for qualifying for health insurance coverage for bariatric surgery. Each insurance com-pany is different, and their set of criteria and processes vary widely. If you have health insurance, I would encourage you to cover your bases by trying to qualify for approval for coverage while also looking into self-payment options.

My employer's plan excluded bariatric surgery coverage, so I decided to find a way to self-pay. I also chose to investigate supplemen-tal insurance, because if you have a surgery that is performed outside regular medical insurance coverage and a complication arises, your regular medical insurance won't cover that cost either. For example, if you had a medically necessary knee surgery with a covered doc-tor and surgical facility, your medical insurance would likely cover a large portion of the costs (initial doctor visit, the surgeon and surgi-cal staff, anesthesiologist, medications, lab work, the operating room, and the hospital stay). Your insurance would also likely cover your post-operative appointments and would pay for the costs if any com-plications (like a blood clot) arose.

But if you've self-paid and a serious complication arises during or after surgery, chances are your medical insurance company won't pay for this either, as the initial surgery was not authorized/covered. That possibility was very scary to me; I am generally a risk-averse person, so the thought of having a serious complication that could bankrupt me and my family worried me for months. Finally, I decided to pay for sup-plemental insurance from a privately held company called Leavitt Risk Partners, offering BLISCare, which provides supplemental coverage for more than 180 procedures across eleven specialties, including bariatric surgery (there are a couple other insurance companies that offer similar coverage). The surgeon and surgical facility must be approved by Leavitt Risk Partners, but it's a fairly straightforward process to get registered. If the doctor you are interested in isn't registered, they can work to pass all tests to qualify. It took less than a week for my surgeon to get qualified.

Both my surgeon and Leavitt Risk Partners helped me to select the specific medical complications that I wanted covered. I chose a protection plan that covered cardiopulmonary thromboembolism, bleeding, infection, leak, perforation, and stenosis/stricture. I then selected the length of time that I wanted coverage in each area. My doctor recommended that, for some of these complications, like cardiopulmonary thromboembolism, I only needed coverage for ninety days. Others, like stenosis/stricture, he recommended keeping for thirty-six months.

Once you select what you want covered and for how long, you pay Leavitt Risk Partners or a similar insurance company up front. I chose a lot of coverage—I probably overdid it, actually—but better safe than sorry. As with all insurance, the best that you can hope for is that you throw your money away and never have to use it. The whole thing cost me an additional $2,000. For me, it was worth the peace of mind.

Cut Gut Organization

I was incredibly fortunate to be able to cover the cost of both the surgery and supplemental insurance. Not everyone is so lucky. As I handed the administrator at the bariatric clinic my credit card, I couldn't help but think of the methadone clinic, where I'd learned that the general public is not very sympathetic to heroin addicts. Addicts, who are already so greatly burdened by their disease, often also have to find a way to fund treatment, and if they are lucky enough to have health insurance in the first place, treatment facilities don't always accept it. This is a main reason so many can't get the help they need.

Most people would support you (at least philosophically if not financially) if you started a nonprofit to raise money for hungry children or homeless puppies. But not everyone will get behind a nonprofit for heroin addicts. They're just not as cute, for one. But more significantly, most people continue to blame addicts for their problems. The same goes for the obese.

All this is to say there's a good chance you will have to pay a significant amount of money out of pocket. That is why I've started Cut Gut Organization to help fund those in need. Cut Gut Organization is a nonprofit on a mission to help prevent disease, improve health, and promote sustainable weight loss by subsidizing some of the costs associated with bariatric surgery. Our vision is to be the leader in providing grants to support individuals to achieve good health and sustained weight loss through bariatric surgery. Cut Gut Organization differentiates itself by lowering barriers of participation and allowing anyone in need to apply (not just those who live below the poverty line or cannot qualify for a personal loan). We believe that being gainfully employed and earning a living should be honored and not lower your chances of qualifying for financial assistance. We want to help those who help themselves.

To find out more about Cut Gut Organization, visit www.cutgut.org.

Cut to the Chase

Let's say you've worked through all of your questions, have a plan for how you will pay for your surgery, learned about necessary preparations, and have (at least to an acceptable degree) overcome your underlying fears about bariatric surgery, and you are now ready to move forward with the surgery. You've had a medical examination (probably more than one), lab tests, an upper endoscopy, an EKG and pulmonary assessment, biometric assessments, and a nutritional assessment. But your presurgery journey is not over yet. Now there are other things to be concerned about. It is time for your psychological evaluation.

The psychological evaluation is a critical part of your own emotional prep. It also helps surgeons to be sure that their patients recognize the seriousness of the operation. Before my surgery, I was required to undergo a ninety-minute session to discuss any questions or concerns that I had and also to verify that I understood the procedure would be irreversible. I was lukewarm on the meeting—not because I don't think that speaking with a psychologist is valuable but because I didn't have much to say, and as a busy executive, mother, and wife, I felt my time was precious and I didn't really want to spend it in a therapist's office. Plus, I knew what I wanted, so what was the point? I thought I could wrap up the session in two sentences: "I have been overweight most of my adult life, my health is starting to be affected, and for many years every diet has failed me. I have done in-depth research on bariatric surgery as I want to live a long healthy life, and I believe this is the path, the only path, to get me there." I decided my mission was to quickly convince the psychologist—let's call her Linda—that I was of sound mind and body and that I understood fully what I was getting into.

With this in mind, you can imagine how surprised I was when the ninety minutes were up and I not only had gotten a lot of solid information out of our conversation but also was thoroughly engaged. There are a few things from the session that stand out in my memory and that helped me tremendously both before and after surgery.

"Post-bariatric surgery life is like life as a new parent," Linda told me.

What the hell does that mean? I thought. "What do you mean?" I asked politely.

"People always tell new parents, 'Your life is really going to change. You have no idea exactly what you are getting into. Your priorities, your time, your relationships are going to be drastically different.' Right?"

"Sure," I said. "That was true in my experience."

"Exactly," Linda said. "Soon-to-be new parents often nod and think, Sure, yeah, I know. But do they? Of course not. *You can only know once you get there.*"

"What do you hope will change post-surgery and post-weight loss?" she asked me.

"Nothing," I said proudly, "other than being healthier." I was proud because the younger me would have said, "A modeling career, new-found riches, gorgeous, loving people surrounding me, the adoration of the masses." OK, I probably wouldn't have said that, or at least not out loud, but I probably would have thought some version of it. In my late forties, however, I truly loved my life. I loved my wonderful family, my loving friends, my adorable four-legged creatures, and my job. Living a longer and healthier life was truly my top priority.

But instead of Linda exclaiming, "You are the perfect surgical candidate; this meeting is concluded!" and pinning a gold star to my shirt, she frowned slightly. "If no change beyond being healthier is what you hope for," she said, "then you're going to be disappointed. People will react to you differently when you're 80 to 100 pounds lighter. And it won't all be positive."

"What do you mean?" I asked.

"Don't get me wrong—you'll likely get a fair amount of positive feedback. That might feel strange in its own way. Men who might not have noticed you or weren't attracted to you before might start acting differently toward you, for better or worse. And women who liked you when you were heavy might feel threatened. I hate to say it, but I have met with women who, after the surgery, found out that some people were their friends in part because they were the 'token fat girl' who made everyone else feel better about themselves. Have you heard of the acronym DUFF?"

"No . . . ," I said hesitantly.

"It's a horrible, horrible term that means 'designated ugly fat friend.'"

My jaw dropped.

"I know, I know, my jaw dropped when I heard it too. Unfortunately, it's a real thing, and *you will find out who your real friends are once you drop the weight.* Then there are the friends who are heavy and felt you were in it together—they might feel betrayed or like you no longer fit in with them. Your family too: your kids, their friends and parents, have viewed you one way, and that'll have to change. Your spouse, your sister, and even your parents might start acting differently."

"They'll be happy for me," I said.

"Of course they will," Linda said. "But think about it: if you were always the heavier sister or daughter, it'll be a big change for them and how they think about their own identity. So if there's any latent jealousy, it could come to the surface. Your relationships with your boss and colleagues could change too. The changes are not necessarily good or bad, but you can count on things being very different.

"Losing weight is not the magic solution for all of life's problems," she said. I pondered her statement for a minute. I suppose it is easy to believe that if you are at a normal body mass index all of your struggles will disappear and be replaced with a huge social circle filled with happiness and adoration, wealth, and high self-esteem that makes you unstoppable.

"You will still have to deal with underlying issues of self-perception and self-esteem—those don't evaporate overnight, no matter what your body looks like. You'll have to deal with negative feelings, and you can't use food to comfort yourself in the same way you have in the past, or blame your weight for your problems.

"Many Americans have surpassed the bottom rungs on Maslow's Hierarchy of Needs, the search for food and shelter and other survival basics, so we've found other things to occupy our time, namely, the pursuit of happiness. So many magazines, social media, self-help books, and TV shows are geared toward either showing you how to increase your happiness or showing you a bunch of people who appear to be much happier than you are. We're just not comfortable with being discontent. Not only that, but we are taught that the slightest feeling of discomfort should prompt immediate action. If you practice this modus operandi, post-surgery is going to be grueling. The surgery you've chosen is not reversible. There will be pain involved, and there will be times you'll feel frustrated because you can no longer consume the amount or types of food that you once did."

She let that sink in for a moment. It is hard to imagine what life will be like with a tiny stomach, and it was true that I'd tended to think more about benefits than drawbacks.

"When you're feeling frustrated, you'll need to *not* act," Linda continued. "You'll have to sit with it, as well as other challenging emotions like sadness, regret, or even despair. *Don't run from uncomfortable emotions.* Sitting with them, really feeling them, is not such a bad thing. It'll give you strength and a better capacity for reflection. It'll show you that pain won't cause you to wither away and die. Ironically, being OK with feeling unhappy can increase your overall happiness."

"Well, I can tell you that, as a global commuter, I spend a big portion of my life sitting on airplanes," I said. "So sitting with discomfort is something I can do."

"Good. Still, I recommend that, before surgery, *you make a list of things you can do if you do find yourself needing an escape, a list of things that make you happy.* Light a candle, make some tea, call a friend, or work on a hobby; do something, anything, you enjoy."

"I appreciate that you did not say 'exercise' as a substitute for food," I told her. "I had a primary care doctor tell me years ago that when I felt like eating something sweet, simply do ten jumping jacks instead, and I'd always be healthy. It is sort of like telling an alcoholic that if they feel like having a drink to just drink a glass of water instead—ridiculous! Yes, you should exercise to maintain health, but I'd like to identify things that I truly enjoy doing, and at this point, exercise is certainly not at the top of the list."

"*You'll also have to make a conscious effort to check in with yourself and examine what you need and what you are feeling and then communicate those things to the people around you.*" A big mistake patients make is not communicating what they need from others. People who love and care about you will try to support you, but they are not mind readers and often do not know what you need. To make it more complicated, what you need the first week post-surgery is often very different than what you will need at month 3 and month 33. To illustrate her point, Linda told me the following story:

A longtime married couple, Jennifer and David, had come to her office for an emergency counseling appointment. She had first met Jennifer twelve months earlier for her presurgical consultation, and they'd spoken by phone six months after that to check in on how Jennifer was doing post-surgery. Jennifer reported that she was doing well. But Jennifer had called out of the blue to ask for an emergency session. She was thinking of leaving David, her husband of twenty-three years, because he was driving her crazy with his daily interrogation about how much weight she'd lost.

When the couple arrived at her office, Jennifer immediately excused herself to use the restroom. Linda turned to David, introduced herself, and then asked, "How's it going?"

Much to her surprise, David said, "Great! Today is Jennifer's one-year surgery anniversary. She tried so many diets before, and she used to get really angry with me because I didn't take more of an interest in how her weight loss was progressing. So I promised myself that I would be more supportive after she woke up from surgery by asking her every day how much weight she has lost. I even set a timer on my watch to remind me." With a huge, genuine smile, David said, "I feel that I am finally giving her the support that she needs."

"Jennifer returned to the room then and expressed her profound irritation with David's behavior," Linda told me.

I laughed. I'd been in situations like this too, mostly at work, playing mediator between a manager and employee. Both individuals would have the best of intentions, but somewhere along the way, they'd miscommunicate or make false assumptions about each other's expectations and things would sour. I realized that I would have to stay conscientious in communicating my changing needs to my family post-surgery.

"David was well meaning," I said. "But I can see why that irritated Jennifer."

"I am happy to report I was able to help them work it out," Linda finished. "I encouraged Jennifer to better communicate exactly the kind of support she needed from David."

Then Linda gave me the most powerful suggestion of all: to *ask for cards of encouragement*. She suggested that, several weeks before my scheduled surgery, I ask those closest to me to write five to ten 3-by-5-inch note cards telling me

- why this surgery is important and the right decision for me; and
- what my having bariatric surgery means to them.

"When you wake up after surgery, you are probably going to ask yourself, 'Oh my gosh, what the hell was I thinking? I should never have done this!' And with all the anesthesia and medication, you will likely not be thinking clearly. It is at those times that the messages from your loved ones will be of utmost help; they will remind you that after years of struggle, you made the right decision."

I didn't realize it at the time, but this would turn out to be one of the most meaningful pieces of advice I'd ever received.

No Guts, No Glory

I did months of research; interviewed nearly a hundred patients, surgeons, clinics, and hospitals; found the "One"; jumped through all the necessary presurgery hoops; and bought supplemental insurance. Dr. Matthew Weiner's practice was in a suburb of Detroit, and though it was slightly more expensive and complicated to have the surgery done out of state (and I was a bit anxious about the logistics, particularly the trip back home), the journey was well worth it. My husband and I traveled 1,924 miles as the crow flies, and I thought to myself, *This will be the last time that I wear one of these damn full-body compression sleeves on a plane.* I was almost nostalgic—almost.

My husband, daughter, son, mother, father, and sister all delivered sealed envelopes to me several weeks before my surgery. I'd left these cards of encouragement untouched, wanting to wait until after the surgery to read them. But the night before, while sitting alone and hungry in my hotel room while my husband was out filling some post-surgery antinausea prescriptions for me (you can't eat much for twenty-four hours before the operation), I unexpectedly went into a presurgery *Oh my god, what am I doing!?* panic. I locked myself in the bathroom and opened the envelopes, one by one, careful not to tear or bend them. I spent nearly two hours reading and rereading them, my family's words of joy and encouragement, their hopes and dreams for me, and their humor. A couple of them had even glued pictures of us onto their notes. I sobbed when I read about their love and worry for me, how important I am to them, and that they cannot imagine a world without me. They told me things I never knew they thought or felt. I felt incredibly special and loved.

I have read those cards of encouragement a thousand times since then. They carried me through that moment and many hard moments since. After reading them for the first time in the hotel bathroom, there was absolutely no doubt that this—bariatric surgery—was the way forward. Here are just a few of them:

You will increase your life expectancy by 10 years. (That's actually a benefit for me!)

I will be with you every step of the way and do whatever it takes for you to be successful !!!

You have chosen the best doctor!

No more high blood pressure. stronger heart!

Jamie,
You have certainly done your
homework on this decision!
No rushing in and hoping. At
first I had doubts, but your
thorough explanation of the logic
in your decision convinced me
that you've made the right
choice here.
　　　　　　Your Loving Dad

The past is gone. Today is full of possibilities.
With each breath you will be aware of the
strength at hand.

I love you with my whole heart.
And with my whole heart, I say thank
you. Thank you for doing this. I know
you will be happier, healthier, more
agile & confident - not to mention your
longevity. I say thank you because
I want all this FOR you! And nothing
makes me happier than when my sissy is
happy. YOU GOT THIS　I ♡ you!

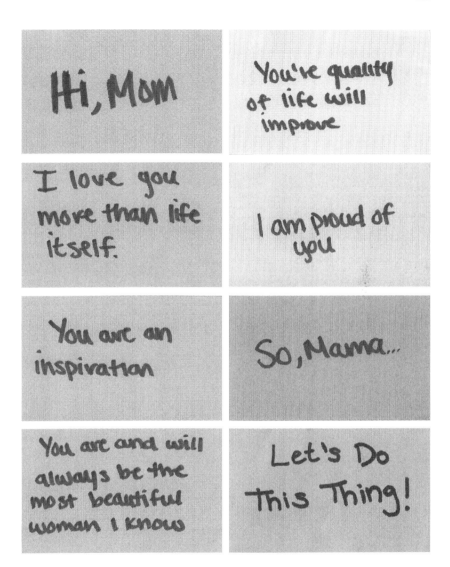

The next morning, as I laid on the gurney being wheeled to the operating room, I felt cold, nervous, and excited. The anesthesiologist came in and talked calmly to me as he did his magic. And then I began to count backward: 10, 9, 8 . . .

CHAPTER 9

Got Cut

Life is like riding a bicycle. To keep your
balance you must keep moving.
—Albert Einstein

The days following the surgery were a bit of a blur. Overall, I didn't have much pain, and my doctor made sure I did not feel nauseated or dizzy. I took a grand total of one pain pill post-surgery. I'd just had 80 percent of my stomach removed, and I felt basically OK. The miracles of modern medicine!

In the hospital, I was immediately able and encouraged to drink water and eat ice chips and within twenty-four hours was discharged from the hospital and given my doctor's blessing to recover in the privacy of my hotel room. Soon I was gingerly taking sips of water and protein shake and slowly pacing the hallways of the hotel to get my body moving and my blood flowing. While I think I would have generally been fine on my own (with the exception of the drive upon discharge from the hospital), I was thankful that my husband had agreed to make the trip with me. I appreciated that he was there to watch over me and extend a loving hand to hold as I took my first few sips and steps.

I wasn't entirely pain free: I had a sore throat from the intubation and, on my right side, a pulling sensation due to the angle the stitches went in as I was laying on the operating table, as well as some occasionally sharp pains. Concerned about the intermittent sharp pains, I called my doctor, who patiently reminded me that pain in the right side or upper back/shoulder is a common symptom after many kinds of surgeries. Air that's pumped into your abdomen during the procedure to make the laparoscopy easier sometimes gets trapped under the ribcage and shoulder. "Don't worry," he said. "That will pass on its own soon enough." And within a couple days, it did.

My mission in life those first few days was to stay hydrated. The order of importance was (1) hydration; (2) protein intake (via liquid protein shakes); and (3) bariatric vitamins (chewable form). Dr. W had explained that hydration at this point in my recovery was vastly more important than protein or vitamins. It's interesting how a physical trauma can narrow your focus to a pinpoint; all I really did those first few days was sleep, drink, and hobble up and down the hotel hallway. And I also spent a lot of time worrying about the plane ride home. I had had surgeries before: C-section, gallbladder removal, and hysterectomy (all due to the effects of my pregnancies and childbirth—it's a darn good thing I have such great kids!). I knew the myriad of possible post-surgery complications, including anesthesia hangover, pain, soreness, swelling, restlessness, constipation, and nausea, not to mention the risk of more serious ones, like a blood clot or internal bleeding. How would I do on the long car rides to and from the airports? What would I do if I began feeling extremely ill on the five-hour-plus plane ride home? I played a "what if" game in my head and probably drove my husband nuts going through every scenario I could imagine.

Three days post-surgery on a sunny cold morning, my husband drove us to the airport in our rental car. I sat reclined in the passenger seat, looking out the window at the sparse white clouds passing overhead. As I've mentioned, I have a complicated long-term relationship with air travel. I suspect most people do, but overweight people do even more so. The flight would be five hours and, being warned about how difficult it would be for me to sit up for that long, I'd splurged on a first-class ticket so I could recline back and take up a little extra room. It turned out I needn't have worried (isn't that usually the way?). The flight was uneventful, and I was back home in no time.

Once home, I found myself wanting a little extra attention, to be waited on by my family. I thought, *When else would I get an excuse to fully indulge in idleness?* But the secret truth was I felt great! The worst part was over, and healing was underway. While my doctor had advised me to take two weeks off work, I only ended up taking one week, and it would have likely been even less if I'd had my surgery done locally. I was back to work the following Monday.

My surgery wasn't public knowledge at this point. And it was fairly easy not to mention it: by all appearances, I hadn't changed. I'd told only a couple trusted colleagues at work. I just wasn't sure if I'd receive the same kind of support I would have if I'd had a different type of surgery, such as a rotator-cuff repair or a thyroidectomy.

I had also thought I'd hidden my weight pretty well (looking back, this was a delusion that helped me cope). I think that, on some level, I felt that in telling everyone about my surgery, I'd be spilling my great big secret that I was seriously overweight. Such was my delusion. I also thought people might think I was ill or depressed. I wasn't interested in anyone's judgy thoughts. On top of all that, I'd been concerned about the risks to my employment if my "elective" surgery were to have gone wrong.

I did, however, tell my boss and two other colleagues whom I trusted. To my utter shock, one of those three had also scheduled the same surgery the day before mine! I was truly stunned to find this out, and I was overjoyed to have someone with whom to compare notes. Presurgery she and I were at a very similar body mass index (BMI). Post-surgery it was really nice to have someone at work to talk to and learn from. I think it helped us both normalize the experience. She tells me frequently that she is doing great, and by all appearances she is. She has told me numerous times that she is very happy with her decision to have bariatric surgery.

Short Cuts: There Are None

Maybe most of all, I was afraid people would think I was taking the easy way out with bariatric surgery. I worried about this not just with my colleagues but also with my kids, both of whom can probably recite my soap-box speech about laziness: how laziness is one of the qualities I dislike most, how we need to work hard and persevere, how my children come from a long line of strong individuals and their direct ancestors worked hard and were mentally tough, and how they survived the trials and tribulations of war, famine, and long and dangerous journeys. And here I was, Ms. Hard Work and Perseverance, not able to work hard enough, persevere enough, to lose weight. If I was preaching against laziness but "taking the easy way out," that would make me a hypocrite. Worse than that, I was someone who was willing to endanger her life for the sake of a so-called quick fix. What if something had happened to me and I hadn't made it out of surgery? What would my children think of me then? What would they tell their children? Would they put "Here lies Jamie J. Palfrey, beloved wife, mother, and hypocrite who died trying to take the easy way out" on my tombstone?

It turns out, these awful thoughts were all just in my mind—my kids have been nothing but supportive throughout this process and have thanked me for taking my life back. Anyone who knows anything about bariatric surgery is not going to think it's a cop-out. (Anyone who knows anything about any kind of surgery is not going to think it is a cop-out; the intimidating phrase *going under the knife* is used for a reason.) I doubt there are many obese people who go into bariatric surgery thinking it will be easy and the weight will just fly off and stay off without effort. Most obese people know all too well how ephemeral weight loss can be and are under no false illusions that the surgery will cure everything without requiring a lifetime commitment to healthy living. Qualified candidates have to stick to a very difficult presurgical diet (covered in chapter 7), and the post-surgery diet is no easier. The presurgical diet had been challenging for me because I was hungry and my ghrrrelin was still working in full effect. The post-surgery diet was challenging, not because I was hungry, weak, or had any type of real cravings, but because I was completely relearning how to eat again.

After my first post-operative appointment, my doctor advanced my diet to include real food—soft things at first like yogurt and apple-sauce or anything blended. Over the next months, my diet continued to advance, first to blended soups and well-cooked vegetables, then to beans and eggs. The next big milestones were nuts and fish, and finally, the ultimate victory: chicken. Slowly, one food at a time, one teaspoon at a time, I made sure whatever I was eating didn't cause pain, nausea, or vomiting. Following this post-surgery diet regime helps ensure your safety and comfort, and aids in breaking the cycle of old eating habits. It also gives your newly rearranged cut gut a chance to heal and learn how to function in a completely different way. *Be patient* and don't rush things—it's not a contest! Depending on the type of bariatric surgery you decide to have, for the rest of your life you should

- avoid or limit alcohol;
- monitor your fluid intake to make sure you are properly hydrated;
- chew foods thoroughly;
- avoid drinking thirty minutes before and after every meal;
- manage your lean protein intake;
- avoid sugars and unhealthy fats;
- take a daily bariatric multivitamin; and
- exercise regularly.

Learning how to eat differently, consuming a fraction of what you once ate, being vigilant about taking vitamins, and avoiding foods and drinks you used to love—that's not easy. Letting go of old routines and habits and exercising regularly—that's not easy either. Sacrificing social norms for the sake of your diet—that can really be tough. Having to deal with boredom, depression, or anxiety without using food—no easy button there either. When it comes to obesity, there is no quick fix, no easy way out. There are no shortcuts.

Am I Cut Out for This?

I had my surgery in September, one month after my fiftieth birthday. The first month after, I focused on staying hydrated and getting enough liquid protein and vitamins. As soon as I could, I started power walking, with a goal of ten thousand steps a day. That first month I lost 18 pounds.

The craziest thing about this period: I was not hungry. This was to be expected, but still I was not prepared for the experience of it. I'd been hungry my whole life, and so much of my time had been focused on food or, more accurately, dieting and avoiding food. But now I just wasn't motivated by food, which felt like a liberation. For the first time in years, my body was recognizing my obesity for what it was: a signal to eat less and move more. Finally, with the surgery having "reset" my set point, my glass Wonkavator floated down from Mount Everest. On a successful day I managed to get 600 calories down. I had to be careful to make sure the calories that I was able to consume were quality (not empty carbohydrates), with high levels of vitamins and minerals, since my new stomach had a lower capacity for nutrient absorption.

I was still nowhere near being able to eat "normally" when my favorite holiday, Halloween, arrived. You may have guessed that my favorite holiday had little to do with the holiday itself but rather the candy! I was still fragile, finding my way back to eating solid food again, and it was the first Halloween in recorded history that I did not eat *any* sweets. I did miss the ritual of it—that certain magical smell that can only be created by throwing a bunch of different types of candy together in a huge plastic pumpkin or pillowcase. I swear, if I closed my eyes and you put a kid's filled Halloween bag under my nose, I would recognize it instantly! There is no other smell like that in the world; it kicks off happy childhood memories of my parents making homemade Darth Vader and R2-D2 costumes for me and my sister, and them holding our hands as we tromped around the neighborhood collecting Reese's Peanut Butter Cups, bite-sized coconutty Almond Joys, Mr. Goodbars, and strawberry- and grape-flavored Fun Dip candies.

The Halloween after my surgery, I could recognize that same smell in my kids' stash, but it just no longer moved me. It didn't fill me with want. In fact, I was filled instead with an overwhelming sense of relief when I realized I had no desire whatsoever to gorge on candy. It was the first October 31 in memory that I actually lost weight.

The Thanksgiving holiday followed quickly thereafter, as it always does, and I made the usual meal for my family: turkey, potatoes (both mashed and baked), fluffy yams with marshmallows, peas, corn, gelatinous cranberry sauce out of the can, and buttery rolls with lots of strawberry jam. None of these foods had passed my lips since I'd gotten my brand-new stomach two months prior. I had been working with my doctor on slowly introducing new foods, and none of these had made it on the list yet. I was doing really well, following the post-operative diet to a T. But on this day I just really wanted *real* food to celebrate with my family. I could only eat 2 tablespoons' worth, so I served myself wee portions of everything. I took my time, chewing slowly, savoring every tiny bite. I was enjoying my family's holiday mood but also paying close attention to stop when I felt full. In spite of my best efforts, I became overly full and did not feel at all well after ingesting food that my body wasn't ready for. Then, an hour after we had finished and my feeling of fullness had greatly diminished, came dessert . . .

I served a few different classic Thanksgiving pies—I love to bake, and I love to watch my husband and kids enjoy what I've made—pumpkin pie, pecan pie, apple pie, and cherry pie. My husband and kids had a couple different kinds, with healthy scoops of vanilla ice cream on top. I served myself a meagre piece of cherry pie, nothing more than a sliver. I took three itty-bitty bites.

Now, most people overeat on Thanksgiving—it's an American tradition. We *brag* about how much we ate, how many different kinds of stuffing and slices of pie we had, and how we ate until our stomachs hurt. Most people can deal with the discomfort by lying on the couch with their belts undone while watching the football game or going for a walk around the block to get some fresh air.

This was not an option for me. Within ten minutes of those three bites, I was sweating, with an incredible pain in my stomach and a full-on anxiety attack ramping up. I left the table and went to my bedroom to be alone with the agony. I knew two things: throwing up for the first time since surgery was likely imminent, and I had probably caused myself a leak—a break in the lining between staples and therefore a break in the boundary between the inside of the stomach and the other internal organs. Stomach acid leaking into my abdominal cavity would be a life-threatening event. And you need to have a CT scan, chest X-ray, and blood count test to officially diagnose it, procedures not so easy to come by on Thanksgiving.

I sobbed from the pain and terror I was feeling. I paced around my bed, in too much pain to lie down, bouncing back and forth in my head between bargaining with God and having an imaginary conversation with my doctor. I begged the universe to forgive me. I felt deep shame as I thought about how far I'd come, with so many people believing in me and helping me along the way. My doctor had laid out exactly what to do and what not to do—and I'd fucked it all up! *You did what?* I imagined my doctor saying, shaking his head. I tried on every excuse. *I was so careful!* I would tell him. *I'm only human, for goodness sake!* followed by *It was the pie!* Still, in my mind, he wagged his finger, tsk-tsking at me. *What did you expect?* I imagined him asking in an accusatory tone.

In real life, my doctor would never tsk-tsk, or wag his finger, for that matter. After two agonizing hours, the prayers must have won out because the extreme nausea subsided, the pain was gone, the dreaded vomiting never came, and my body seemed to return to normal. I knew then that I had not caused a leak, and I vowed on all that was holy that I would never, ever push my new stomach that way again.

If you get "cut," your body has to learn how to digest and process even the most basic foods again, like a baby going from mother's milk to solid foods. You will have to be patient and take things slowly as you get to know your new stomach or intestines. I still try to visualize my new little stomach as precious and tender. I remind myself that the little bit of tissue left is working hard to do everything that the whole stomach used to. It takes some time for it to learn what to do. It needs food well chewed and mindfulness around what/how much is coming "down the pike." If you get gastric bypass, this applies to your "new" intestines too. Be kind to them, because they are working hard for you. They are all that you've got or will ever have, and their job of breaking down and properly digesting nutrients to keep you alive and healthy is of no small importance. I fought my body for so many years. It has been a remarkable experience learning how to be thoughtful and kind to it.

Spill Your Guts:
To Tell or Not to Tell?

Two weeks after the Thanksgiving fiasco, I had an opportunity to test my promise to the universe. For the first time post-surgery, I ventured to a restaurant to celebrate a birthday with some friends. Still fearful and delicate, I had a mini-panic attack as I looked over the menu, remembering what I used to order at this popular Asian infusion: a glass of tannin-rich cabernet, the chicken lettuce wrap appetizer followed by gluten-free Mongolian beef with white rice and a decadent no-flour chocolate cake with raspberry purée dessert. What should I order now? What if I overordered? What if I ate something that didn't agree with me and there I was, miles from home? Would my friends, who were unaware that I'd had surgery, think I was rude if I did not eat?

To be honest, I didn't enjoy the birthday dinner very much. I don't think I ate even one bite, making a weak excuse about the food being too salty. Afterward, my husband said I'd been unusually quiet and a bit snappy when I got home that night. He had no idea what I had been going through. At the end of the day, I was actually quite proud of myself for managing my internal drama and not repeating Thanksgiving. Even though the experience was a struggle, I continued to feel strong about my decision to have bariatric surgery. I saw at every turn that this was *not* an easy way out!

This situation was the first of many in which I had to find a way to eat almost nothing *and* deal with the social ramifications. So much of family and community life revolves around food. The birthday cake, the Christmas spread, and hot dogs and hamburgers on the Fourth of July—these occasions are as much about food as they are about particular stories or celebrations. Building trust and rapport with colleagues or clients usually involves cocktails, coffee, or a shared meal; they call it "breaking bread" for a reason. Would I be able to not eat "normally" but maintain normal social connections?

I did my research. On a YouTube video, a fellow bariatric patient suggested that if you go to someone's house for dinner, just tell them that you accidentally already ate. This had apparently worked well for her, but to me it sounded silly, bordering on rude. Who would be so thoughtless as to eat beforehand, knowing full well that the host had made dinner?

We all have to find our own way down the post-surgery path, deciding how much we want to disclose and to whom. Going out to a restaurant is a great way to practice this tricky conversation, because it's unlikely the server will be personally offended if you don't finish your meal. At least, they won't be personally offended as long as you tip well. Here's how it usually happens for me:

The waiter begins to clear the plates. When she gets to mine, which still contains one-half to three-quarters of the Caesar salad or vegan bean soup that I ordered, she pauses. Invariably the waiter says, "Did you not like your meal?"

"I liked it very much; it was delicious," I reply, a smile on my face.

The waiter looks confused. "OK . . . well, then would you like a box to take it home?"

"Oh, no, thank you, but I appreciate the offer," I say politely. Then I'll tip them the usual 20 percent.

Now, don't get me wrong, I am not out to waste food or money. In fact, I don't eat out often anymore, preferring to cook at home, where my family has fully accepted my new eating protocol. I have even bought myself a colorful and fun "mini" set of dishes and silverware that I use at every meal to remind myself of my best portion sizes and to feel I am filling my plate and utensil. When I do go out to eat, I try to split appetizers or entrées with other people, or I just have a couple bites of theirs. If I really want my own thing, I've learned to eat what is healthy and comfortable and then stop, without feeling guilty or making excuses.

But rest assured that, no matter how smooth or friendly your explanation or redirection, people will question you. It took me months to start to tell people that my change in eating habits and weight loss was due to bariatric surgery, and the number I told was small. For the first year post-surgery, I often straight-up lied about why I was barely eating (mostly to strangers). I said things like I wasn't feeling well or something was wrong with the food. Every once in a great while, someone would push me about it, and I would tell them that I had bariatric surgery and therefore could not eat much. Often, they would be speechless; most people don't really know what to say or how to process the information. Sometimes they'd say, "Oh, OK, well, that's nice," then change the subject. Every once in a while, someone would say, "I've thought about doing that too, but I didn't think I was a candidate. Can you tell me more about it?"

I wrote this book for both groups of people—those who are brave enough to talk openly about it and those who are eager to change the subject. We praise people who lose weight through sweat and starvation (because of the obvious grit and willpower involved). But for most of us with a metabolic disease, substantial and sustainable weight loss is as much about grit as it is about addressing the disease itself head on. Unfortunately, bariatric surgery is not yet a badge of honor like surviving brain cancer, and I still struggle with admitting to it sometimes. Writing this deeply personal book has been hard at times. I am finally pulling off the veil. It has become incredibly important to me that the millions of Americans who meet the criteria for bariatric surgery be aware of its lifesaving and positive life-changing effects. Perhaps I owe it to them (and myself) to get a T-shirt that says "BODY AND LIFE COMPLIMENTS OF BARIATRIC SURGERY!"

Whether it's prompted by an old acquaintance you bump into at the grocery store or a server at a restaurant who seems irritated by your special requests, you will be faced with the dilemma of whether to tell someone you have had bariatric surgery. For those who know you, the changes in your physical appearance can be shocking. That, coupled with your new eating habits, will lead to some potentially awkward moments. The choice to tell or not to tell is, of course, personal and situational. There are no right or wrong answers here. As I've said before, I hope that someday we'll get to a point where this conversation is no big deal. We now talk openly about subjects that would have been verboten in the past, such as racism, homosexuality, abortion, the gender pay gap, and sexual misconduct in the workplace. So why not obesity as a disease and bariatric surgery as a mainstream treatment?

The people with whom I eat regularly—family, friends, and coworkers—all now know about the surgery. They know I am going to quiz the cook at friends' houses, that even though I'll try to keep it simple at restaurants, every meal will be like that scene out of *When Harry Met Sally*. (Harry: "I'll have a number 3." Sally: "I'd like the chef salad, please, with the oil and vinegar on the side, and the apple pie à la mode . . . but I'd like the pie heated, and I don't want the ice cream on top; I want it on the side. And I'd like strawberry instead of vanilla if you have it. If not, then no ice cream, just whipped cream, but only if it's real. If it's out of a can, then nothing." Sally was ahead of her time.) They are patient if not slightly amused by the predictability of it all.

They also know that I thoroughly enjoy my food even though I'm only able to eat about half as much as I used to.

Though I don't shout it from the rooftops, I am out of the closet. A few months ago, I went to a corporate dinner out of town with people I don't see very often, and at the end of the meal one of my colleagues said, "You didn't like it?"

I used my regular line. "It was delicious," I replied. "I just get full easily."

"Oh, that's right," he said. "You had bariatric surgery." He stopped, his eyes getting wide. "Oh, shoot! Is it OK to say that?" He looked sheepish.

"Yes, it's perfectly fine," I said, smiling.

The Final Cut:
Learning How to Live All Over Again

There are obvious dietary and physical changes that you can expect post-bariatric surgery, such as eating smaller amounts, limiting alcohol, and of course, weight loss. There were also a couple changes that I did not expect:

- *A change in food preferences.* I'd known that my food intake would be limited due to the smaller size of my stomach and the change in metabolic hormones and processes; I was not prepared for my sudden ambivalence toward the foods I'd previously loved. Ice cream, potato chips, and soda just didn't hold the same attraction they once did. Today, it goes beyond ambivalence to aversion, particularly when it comes to ice cream and fried foods. It's not that I can't eat them; it's that they just don't taste that good anymore, and the few times I have taken a bite or two of my son's chocolate ice cream cone or a friend's French fries, I ended up feeling bad physically. The way my body reacts to soda is not so gentle either: one sip and I'll feel like my stomach is going to explode. (By the way, this reaction to carbonation is very uncommon, and most people are fine drinking carbonated drinks post-surgery—just don't drink naturally or artificially sweetened soda, as both are bad for you and highly discouraged post-surgery.) To no longer be pulled toward high-calorie processed foods—that is nothing short of a miracle!

- *Mourning the loss of appetite for formerly favorite foods.* I've had some great times with Sunday morning waffles and Friday night cosmos. Potato chips and double mint chocolate chip ice cream have gotten me through many a hard day. At times I have mourned the loss of these old food friends. But nostalgia can't overcome the messages my body and mind are telling me today. Now I must manage stress or exhaustion in new, healthier ways. Luckily, I have also developed new favorite foods, so all is not lost. I love to eat papaya with a bit of lime juice on it for a treat. This appeals to me much more than a bowl of ice cream. Never in a million years did I think I'd be able to say that with a straight face!

- *The happy surprise of metabolism, hunger, and energy working "normally" again.* For me, it had been thirty years since my metabolism worked as it should! I'd heard stories of people having bariatric surgery and then being able to go off their blood pressure pills almost immediately, or quickly resolving type 2 diabetes or prediabetes, but I had trouble believing them. It just seemed too good to be true. But in the case of bariatric surgery, it is both good *and* true. Something about the surgery seems to have "reset" my body and mind and ended my complex metabolic disease. It is absolutely unbelievable—and real.

Living in Gratitude

The other day, I was griping to my sister over the phone about the amount of travel I've had to do lately. (It's a regular part of my job, and I love meeting new people from all over the world, but every now and then I get homesick and just plain worn out.) She said, "At least you are healthy now!" And she was right. I no longer have to squeeze myself into a full-body compression suit before boarding my flight, and my ankles don't swell up and hang over the tops of my shoes. My seat belt has a good 12 inches to spare. And I no longer receive dirty looks as I make my way down the aisle, but it still irritates me that I and many others have had to endure such openly judgmental behavior.

With the exception of this one conversation with my sister, I do not take my new freedoms in the world or my newfound health for granted. I am amazed by how convenient it is to simply throw on a nice-fitting pair of jeans, normal socks, normal-width shoes, and a small T-shirt and roll out on a Saturday morning. What used to take me forty-five minutes—changing ill-fitting clothes and spending way too long compensating with my hair and makeup (and still loathing the way I looked and felt)—now takes me five minutes. My husband much appreciates this! This certainly doesn't mean that my self-esteem is now tipping the Richter scale or that I don't still have normal struggles and concerns with the way I look from time to time. But I feel more at ease in my skin now. Mostly, I wish I hadn't spent so much time loathing myself in the first place.

Nor will I get used to the fact that now, when I do what I am supposed to, my body responds. My body no longer drives me toward obesity with the force of a hurricane; I can let go of fad diets and health crazes—for the first time in perhaps my whole life, I feel confident in my body's ability to maintain a healthy weight. This is a completely new experience for me, and it is exhilarating.

I cannot afford to get complacent though. Today I weigh myself almost daily. I watch what I eat, and I exercise regularly at home. It's work, but I want to live a long and vital life. And for the first time since I became overweight, I am seeing results from my hard work.

It is hard to talk about post-bariatric surgery life without falling into the "thin is good, fat is bad" trap. I'll admit, I no longer feel like my weight precedes me in every conversation, or assume that people register "she's fat" first and my name second. I feel more comfortable walking into a room, presenting at a meeting, and boarding an airplane. But those who loved me before don't love me any more or any less now. For them, my weight never preceded me, and in retrospect, I wish I hadn't always been so conscious of it, allowing it to affect my every interaction.

I have changed, inside and out. Every once in a while, I'll see my reflection, and instead of having to do a double take, I say to myself, *There is the healthy me! I knew she was in there somewhere.* I'm the same old me—just a more energetic and contented version.

It is important to note that the love and support of my family, friends, and coworkers have had a profound impact on my success through this process. My husband, who has always been a healthy role model for me, has made a huge difference by supporting my changes wholeheartedly. Adapting to life post-surgery would have been infinitely more difficult if I had had negative influences and unsupportive behavior around me.

I am *well* now—and I don't use that word lightly. I am not only physically well but also well in my mind. I feel free of an all-consuming burden, and I am no longer continuously punishing myself. I am light in body, mind, and spirit. To say it's a miracle, to say if I can do it, you can too, sounds disappointingly cliché, but it's true. I am living, breathing proof of hope, health, and enduring change. When nothing upon nothing ever worked, bariatric surgery did. Completely and wholly—it is the best decision I've ever made.

EPILOGUE

When I began my journey of bariatric surgery to reclaim my life and longevity, I didn't set out to write a book about it. And I certainly didn't set out to start a nonprofit organization to help others with fulfilling *their* dream of bariatric surgery. But sometimes life chooses you and changes you in unexpected ways. My newfound health and the ability to give back are beautiful gifts!

> *We delight in the beauty of a butterfly,*
> *but rarely admit the changes it has gone*
> *through to achieve that beauty.*
> —Maya Angelou.

At fifty-two years old, I am finally a healthy and stable 153 pounds as a result of having bariatric surgery. Having gone through years of misleading and incorrect information regarding weight loss and long-term health, I have become impassioned about providing mainstream educational and financial resources to those who want and qualify for this life-changing metabolic surgery. Cut Gut Organization was founded with the idea that anyone with a body mass index of 30 or greater should consider bariatric surgery as a mainstream option for weight loss when diet and exercise have failed. This view moves us away from looking at surgery for weight loss as being reserved for the morbidly obese.

Cut Gut Organization is a nonprofit on a mission to prevent disease, improve health, and promote sustainable weight loss through subsidizing some of the costs associated with bariatric surgery. Our vision is to be the leader in providing grants and education to support individuals in achieving good health and sustained weight loss through bariatric surgery. Cut Gut Organization is one of the only nonprofits in the country that will provide grant assistance to help qualified patients pay for a portion of their bariatric weight-loss surgery.

For more information, please visit www.cutgut.org. Thank you in advance for your support.

RESOURCES

National Heart, Lung, and Blood Institute, www.nhlbi.nih.gov

On Death and Dying, Dr. Elisabeth Kübler-Ross

The Economist, The Caveman's Curse

Diets

Body Love: Live in Balance, Weigh What You Want, and Free Yourself From Food Drama Forever, Kelly Leveque

The Truth about Fat, Anthony Warner

Why Diets Make Us Fat: The Unintended Consequences of Our Obsession with Weight Loss, Sandra Aamodt

Addiction

In the Realm of Hungry Ghosts: Close Encounters with Addiction, Gabor Maté

Unbroken Brain: A Revolutionary New Way of Understanding Addiction, Maia Szalavitz

Culture

Alzheimer's Disease: What If There Was A Cure?, Dr. Mary T. Newport

The Body Is Not an Apology: The Power of Radical Self-Love, Sonya Renee Taylor

Body Love: A Fat Activism Colouring Book, Allison Tunis

Fat Activism: A Radical Social Movement, Charlotte Cooper

Fat Girl on a Plane: A Novel, Kelly deVos

The Feminine Mystique, Betty Freidans

Hunger: A Memoir of (My) Body, Roxane Gay

Shrill: Notes from a Loud Woman, Lindy West

Two Whole Cakes: How to Stop Dieting and Learn to Love Your Body, Lesley Kinzel

You Have Such A Pretty Face, Kelley Gunter

Bariatric Surgery

American Society for Metabolic and Bariatric Surgery, https://asmbs.org

Obesity Action Coalition, www.obesityaction.org

Dr. Matthew Weiner

Movies and Television Shows

Dietland

Dumplin'

I Feel Pretty

Blogs/Bloggers

Alysse Dalessandro, https://readytostare.com

Kelvin Davis, https://notoriouslydapper.com

Jessica Hinkle

Caleb Luna

Cat Polivoda, http://catinspired.com

Bethany Rutter, https://bethanyrutter.com

Ashleigh Shackelford, http://ashleighshackelford.com

Virgie Tovar, www.virgietovar.com

Leah Vernon, www.beautyandthemuse.net

Your Fat Friend

Podcasts

Bad Fat Broads, Ariel Woodson and KC Slack

TEDx Talks

"I Am Fat—How to Be Confident and Love Your Body Size," Victoria Welsby

"Why It's OK to Be Fat," Golda Poretsky

ACKNOWLEDGMENTS

This book was made possible by the millions of people who have steadfastly dieted and exercised as the means to significant and sustainable weight loss and have demonstrated that those methods alone repeatedly fail for most obese people.

Thank you to the men and women, both patient and physician, that have blazed the bariatric surgery trail before me. You have helped pave the way back to health for me and the millions that will come after.

All my love and gratitude to my family whose encouragement has kept me going through all of life's rollercoasters!

Accolades to the medical community and news media for starting to listen, talk about, and take action in supporting bariatric surgery as a lifesaving treatment for obesity. It will take your continued support to break down taboos associated with this remarkable and lifechanging therapy, ultimately helping to make it accessible to the mainstream.

A heartfelt thank you to the amazing team at Girl Friday Productions who've been instrumental to this book's success! Special thanks to Alexander Rigby, the ever-patient publishing manager and project management wizard; Georgie Hockett, a true marketing guru with a brilliant sense of humor; Simone Girrondo, a savvy and skillful editor who is a rare gem of an editor that's actually fun to work with; and Rachel Marek, for creating the beautiful and imaginative cover design!

ABOUT THE AUTHOR

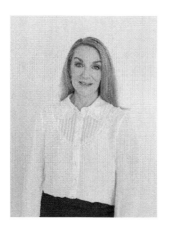

Jamie J. Palfrey earned her master's of education in Human Resources, Occupational Training & Development and Instructional Design from the University of Louisville, Summa Cum Laude. She has worked as a senior human resources leader for more than twenty years. She lives with her husband and two children in Ravensdale (suburb of Seattle), Washington, along with their many farm animals.

Jamie is the president of Cut Gut Organization, a nonprofit on a mission to prevent disease, improve health, and promote substantial and sustainable weight loss for people who have a 30+ BMI by providing grants to subsidize the individual out-of-pocket costs of bariatric surgery. To find out more, please visit www.cutgut.org or contact info@cutgut.org.

Made in the USA
Columbia, SC
16 January 2020